W9-AQZ-822

OUR FAVORITE QUOTES WE SHARE WITH YOU
(you will find them where space allows.)

American people have distinct needs. They have a thinking, unfolding world with which to deal. We feel we all need to be inspired with the words of wisdom of great men who have learned the secrets of the ages.

Life should be very simple, and all the beauty of nature and natural joys we can use are right at hand.

These words of wisdom will appeal to your good common sense! They will guide you in your daily living — for they are practical truths concerning everyday life, from the writings of great minds.

Our goals in life are to seek physical, mental and spiritual perfection. To obtain these priceless blessings we make no compromises and will allow no one or any circumstances to prevent us from attaining these treasures.

— Paul C. Bragg and Patricia Bragg

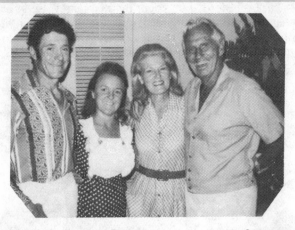

Jack LaLanne, Patricia Bragg, Elaine LaLanne & Paul Bragg

Jack says, "Bragg saved my life at age 14 when I attended the Bragg Health & Fitness Lecture in Oakland, California." From that day on, Jack has lived the health life and teaches Health & Fitness to millions every morning with his T.V. Exercise Show.

HI-PROTEIN

MEATLESS

HEALTH

RECIPES

With History And Reasons

At last! Abundant protein without meat...let your Health Food Store be your meat market and save. Includes recipes for helping to gain and maintain youthfulness. "What-to-do" and "how-to-do-it" information on following the road to vitality. Chapters on hints to vital health, vegetarianism and long-life!

PAUL C. BRAGG N.D., Ph.D.
Life Extension Specialist

PATRICIA BRAGG Ph.D.
Beauty and Diet Expert

Published by
Health Science
Box 477, Desert Hot Springs, California 92240, U.S.A.

HI PROTEIN
MEATLESS
HEALTH RECIPES
With History
and Reasons
By

PAUL C. BRAGG, N.D., Ph.D.
Life Extension Specialist

and
Patricia Bragg

Copyright © Health Science
Second Printing — MCMLXXV

All rights, including the Right of translation into other languages, are reserved by the Publisher. No part of this book may be reproduced in any form, by mimeograph or any other means, without permission in writing from the Publisher.

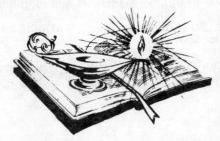

Published in the United States, Australia and England by
HEALTH SCIENCE · Box 477, Desert Hot Springs, California 92240 U.S.A.

Library Of Congress Catalog Card Number: 74-15983
ISBN: 0-87790-030-2

Printed in the United States of America

TOTAL HEALTH FOR THE TOTAL PERSON

In a broad sense, "Total Health for the Total Person" is a combination of physical, mental, emotional, social, and spiritual components. The ability of the individual to function effectively in his environment depends on how smoothly these components function as a whole. Of all the qualities that comprise an integrated personality, a well-developed, totally fit body is one of the most desirable.

A person may be said to be totally physically fit if they function as a total personality with efficiency and without pain or discomfort of any kind. That is to have a Painless, Tireless, Ageless body, possessing sufficient muscular strength and endurance to maintain an effective posture, successfully carries on the duties imposed by the environment, meets emergencies satisfactorily and has enough energy for recreation and social obligations after the "work day" has ended, meets the requirements for his environment through efficient functioning of his sense organs, possesses the resilience to recover rapidly from fatigue, tension, stress and strain without the aid of stimulants, and enjoys natural sleep at night and feels fit and alert in the morning for the job ahead.

Keeping the body totally fit and functional is no job for the uninformed or the careless person. It requires an understanding of the body, sound health and eating practices, and disciplined living. The results of such a regimen can be measured in happiness, radiant health, agelessness, peace of mind, in the joy of living and high achievement.

Paul C. Bragg and Patricia Bragg

FOOD FOR THOUGHT

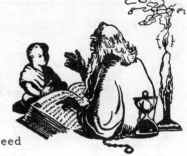

The Great Sin — Fear

The Best Day — Today

The Best Town — Where You Succeed

The Best Work — What You Like

The Best Play — Work

The Greatest Stumbling Block — Egotism

The Greatest Mistake — Giving Up

The Most Expensive Indulgence — Hate

The Greatest Trouble-maker — One Who Talks Too Much

The Most Ridiculous Trait — False Pride

The Most Dangerous Man — The Liar

The Greatest Need — Common Sense

The Greatest Thought — God

The Greatest Wealth — Health

The Greatest Gift You Can Give or Receive — Love

The Greatest Race To Win — A Long Vigorous Life

Man's Greatest Companion and Friend — Good Books

Your Enemies — Envy, Greed, Self-Indulgence, Self-Pity

Life's Greatest Adventure — Growth on the Physical, Mental and Spiritual Plane

Most Disgusting — A Show Off

Most Repulsive — A Bully

Most Overbearing Manner — Arrogance

Man's Greatest Stumbling Block — Ignorance

The Greatest Sieve — Before You Say Anything, Say To Yourself, Is It Kind? — Is It True? — Is It Necessary?

* THE CLEVEREST MAN *

ONE WHO ALWAYS DOES WHAT HE THINKS IS RIGHT

BE A CLEVER MAN!

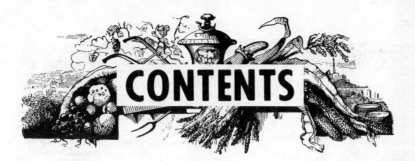

CONTENTS

Contents

Contents

Contents

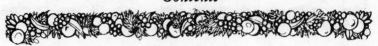

Contents

Contents

Contents

Contents

Contents

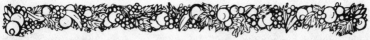

Ponce de Leon,

Searched for the "Fountain of Youth".

If he had only known —

— it's within us...

Created by the food we eat!

"Food can make or break you!"

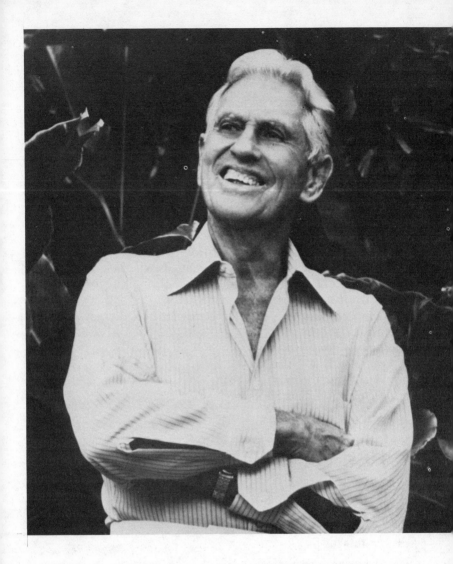

PAUL C. BRAGG, N.D., Ph.D.
Life Extension Specialist

One of the World's Foremost Authorities
on Scientific Nutrition and Physical Fitness.

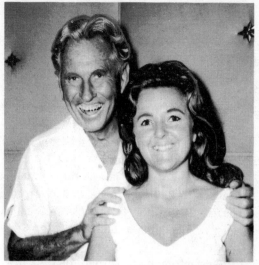

INTRODUCTION

By

PATRICIA
BRAGG

Paul C. Bragg and Daughter Patricia

Go ahead—pick a protein, a vegetable protein preferably. Because in a very few years meat prices may make steaks, chops, roasts and hamburgers seem like gold bullion!

Today many institutions, schools and colleges are experimenting with vegetable proteins to replace the more expensive meat proteins. Today millions of Americans are on vegetarian diets and the numbers will increase rapidly as the price of meat soars to astronomical figures.

In the past, vegetarianism has been practiced mainly by members of religious sects, humanitarians, meatless diet enthusiasts, or by individuals who had some ailment whose treatment required exclusion of meat proteins from the diet.

Today, however, the younger generation considers vegetarianism the "In" thing. They're interested in vegetarianism not only as a health measure and a protest against the exhorbitant price of meat, but also feel that a meatless diet will elevate their consciousness to a higher level.

Recently a noted economist said that the time is not very far off until meat will price itself out of existence, and people will be getting their products from meat analogs (meat-like products) processed from spun fibers of soy protein, wheat, buckwheat, millet and soybeans. Even today, meat analog sales are up $200 million a year.

1

As the Government takes more responsibility in the movement toward vegetable protein, people will realize that one can be fed on a plant diet with great satisfaction and sound, good nutrition.

After all, man's original diet was practically meatless, virtually a lacto-vegetarian diet, and 70% of the world's population today subsists on a diet of which only 5% to 10% of the calories come from animal protein.

If the price of meat is a good reason for switching to vegetarianism today, by A.D. 2050 overpopulation may be the cause for 19 million to switch to vegetarianism, since cattle raising will become a totally inadequate way to produce protein food.

Other factors have turned people toward becoming vegetarians. Meat contains high amounts of saturated fats (cholesterol), uric acid and other toxic materials. These toxins help bring on heart disease, arthritis, gout, kidney and liver trouble.

When my father, Paul Bragg, first advocated meatless or very light meat diets some 60 years ago, it was chiefly because of these inherent toxins in meat itself. In recent decades, however, more and more harmful chemicals have been added to animal products—first in processing, and then in feeding the animals. Cattle especially are fed drugs to accelerate growth and put on weight, and to make matters (or meat) worse they are allowed very little exercise. The result is that these are actually sick animals which are butchered for meat. No wonder that recent medical findings, as reported in the WALL STREET JOURNAL, cite the heavy consumption of beef as a factor in the increase of colon-rectal cancer among Americans.

The idea that meat is essential in the diet is no longer valid. Many outstanding investigators today agree with my father that much better health and longer life may be gained by significantly reducing or even eliminating meat eating. They feel that curtailing the heavy artificial stimulation of the meat proteins will bring greater relaxation, peace of mind, serenity and tranquility throughout the entire body.

When pure rules of business and conduct are observed, then there is true religion.

A vegetarian diet—fortified with lacto-vegetarian proteins such as natural cheese, eggs, yogurt, Brewer's yeast, wheat germ, beans, sprouts, whole cereal grains, avocados, nuts and nut butters, seeds—can form a delicious and nutritious adventure in gourmet meatless cookery. As discussed in this book, natural food supplements serve a healthful purpose in rounding out the vegetarian diet. There are many good vegetable protein and Vitamin B-12 supplements, the two factors that are most often insufficient in a strictly vegetarian diet.

Many arthritics have found great benefit in vegetarianism. Countless numbers of arithritic sufferers have been relieved of pain and agony by turning to the vegetarian diet, and thus cleansing their bodies of accumulated uric acid created by meat. Body chemistry varies so with each individual, that some people create a high uric acid even from light meat intake.

Many vegetarians have testified that by eliminating meat from the diet, they have been relieved of bronchial congestion.

Meat is an acid-forming food, and its digestion requires a large amount of hydrochloric acid. Many people are deficient in hydrochloric acid, and find it difficult to digest meat products. As a consequence, they may suffer from stomach acidity, toxic poison and upset stomach. By changing to a meatless diet, many problems of stomach acidity have shown marked improvement.

Actually, a lacto-ovo-vegetarian diet does not differ markedly from the average American diet. The main difference is that meat is replaced with a variety of legumes, natural cheeses, fertile eggs, Brewer's yeast, wheat germ, nuts and nut butters, seeds, whole grains, meat analogs and vegetables.

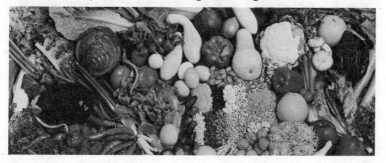

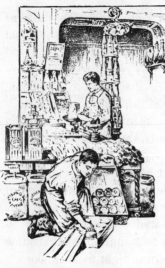

YOUR HEALTH FOOD STORE
CAN SUBSTITUTE FOR YOUR
"MEAT MARKET"

Every person on a vegetarian diet should have his daily ration of Vitamin B-12. This essential nerve vitamin is naturally present in meat, but there is no known practical plant source of B-12 except in sea vegetation such as kelp. (We use kelp seasoning on our food.) Vitamin B-12 is a food supplement which can be purchased in any health food store.

Your health food store can be your meatless butcher shop, as it specializes in meatless foods, organically grown foods, and has a bountiful number of vegetarian products which make for delicious and nutritious eating.

For instance, instead of empty calorie supermarket pasta made from refined white flour ... macaroni, spaghetti, noodles, etc. ... your health food store carries a line of whole wheat and soya pasta made from rich, organically grown grains brimming full of plant proteins. For less than $1.00, you can obtain enough protein—so necessary to optimal nutrition—to feed five people. So go to your health food store and investigate the meatless organic proteins.

The claim of vegetarians that the meatless diet is a means of health improvement and rejuvenation has been borne out by my own experience as a nutritionist. With my father, Paul Bragg, I have traveled extensively throughout the world, and have found hundreds of vegetarians who were radiant with

4

health, and who maintained great strength, endurance and vitality, and seemed to be living in agelessness.

It is unnecessary to kill to eat to live. From the standpoint of health, meat contains the highest bacteria count of any food. In my opinion, a well balanced vegetarian diet allows the body to function on its highest possible level, unhampered by toxic uric acid and other harmful residues built up by meat eating.

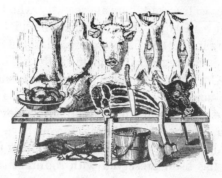

CURED MEATS MAY CAUSE CANCER

Sodium nitrite is a chemical that cures meat, makes it look better, and prevents botulism. But it may also lead to cancer. Pressure is growing to force producers to find an equally effective preservative for meat cured foods such as hot dogs, bologna, salami, lunch meats, pastrami, corned beef, bacon and ham.

For some time it has been known that sodium nitrite is toxic in large doses, and for that reason the Federal Drug Administration has limited its use. But it is only in recent years that medical and scientific research, spearheaded by the School of Medicine at the University of Nebraska, has shown a possible carcinogenic aspect to the danger.

The threat of cancer arises when a nitrite combines with amines, which are part of the make-up of all meats and many other foods. The compound called "nitrosamine" is formed during cooking or perhaps even during the process of digestion. Nitrosamine, when administered in large doses, has caused malignant tumors in experimental animals.

5

Dr. Michael Jacobson, a microbiologist who was educated at the Massachusetts Institute of Technology, urges consumers to avoid all foods containing sodium nitrite. "You won't necessarily die because you eat a piece of bacon," he said, "but there is some small hazard."

In any case, the risks are being studied by the Food and Drug Administration, the Federal Agricultural Department, the meat industry, cancer researchers, Congressional committees and consumer advocates. And there are scientist who think that the high incidence of stomach cancer in Finland is due to the sodium nitrite in smoked fish, so plentiful in the Finnish diet.

A research study recently completed at the Medical School of Loma Linda University in Redlands, California, shows significantly lower incidence of cancer, heart trouble and other degenerative diseases when a meatless diet is followed.

When you eat the vegetarian diet, you have none of the health hazards that one faces when eating either fresh meat or meat which has been preserved with sodium nitrite or other chemical preservatives.

PET OWNERS - BEWARE! Don't feed your dogs and cats food containing sodium nitrite!

Veterinarians are very busy treating sick dogs and sick cats. I have a cousin who is a veterinarian, and I asked him what he thought was the basic cause of so much sickness among dogs and cats.

"Patricia," he said, "practically all canned dog and cat foods are heavily saturated with sodium nitrite, and I believe that this chemical which cures meat causes illness among pets, just as scientists claim that it does with humans.

He told me that pets suffer from heart trouble, strokes, kidney and skin problems, constipation and various other disorders. In outlining diets for dogs and cats, he eliminates all pet foods containing sodium nitrite.

WISDOM DOES NOT show itself so much in precept as in life—a firmness of mind and mastery of appetite. —Seneca.

ANIMAL FATS CAN BE HARMFUL

Dr. Ancel Keys, a celebrated cardiologist, says, "A correlation has been suspected between the instance of heart trouble and a diet rich in animal fats."

The villain is widely identified as cholesterol, a waxy indigestible substance in all animal fats. It is deposited on the walls of the arteries, impeding and sometimes blocking the passage of the blood. This produces excessive strain on the heart to maintain circulation through the constricted arteries. The arteries of the heart itself may become clogged, further impeding its pumping action.

In the same report on cancer research in the WALL STREET JOURNAL, to which I referred earlier, animal and especially beef fat, as well as the meat, has been linked to cancer of the colon and rectum. Thus larded beef, so-called "choice", poses a double threat.

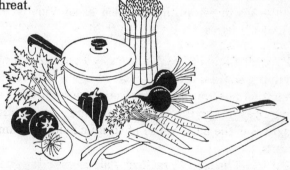

VEGETARIAN GOURMET COOKERY

In my opinion, a vegetarian diet is preferable to a flesh-meat diet for many reasons. It is more humane. . .it is condusive to good health. . .and it is more simple and economical. I believe that a vegetarian diet is essential to our civilization, to universal brotherhood, and to the increase of human happiness.

Well informed nutritional scientists agree that the vegetarian diet is nutritionally adequate. You may exclude most fish, flesh and fowl, and substitute edible raw nuts and seeds of all kinds, legumes such as peas, beans and lentils, whole grain cereals, vegetables, fruit, milk, fertile eggs, natural cheeses, unsalted butter, fats and oils of plant origin, honey, herbs and spices.

It should be obvious from this list that vegetarianism does not mean a diet of merely vegetables. Indeed, the word comes from "vegetus" which means "vigorous."

"But isn't vegetarian cookery a lot of trouble?" you ask.

This question often arises, and the answer is: Neither more nor less trouble than any other kind of nutritious cooking. Truthfully, I find it easier and more interesting. The skillful use of herbs and spices can make it a gourmet adventure. And there are many easily prepared, nutritious and delicious vegetarian meals that require no cooking at all. For example: a protein salad of cottage cheese, tomato, avocado and lettuce, with 100% whole wheat bread and unsalted butter.

Many misinformed people have a dark picture of vegetarianism, and feel that the diet is not tasty or appetizing. But if such people will investigate vegetarian gourmet cookery as given in this book, they will find that the vegetarian diet can be not only health rewarding but also exceptionally nutritious, delicious taste treat.

Yours for Health,

Patricia Bragg

P.S.

Abbreviations Used in These Recipes

tsp	— teaspoon	pt	— pint
tbsp	— tablespoon	lb	— pound
c	— cup	oz	— ounce
qt	— quart		

The best service a book can render is, to impart truth, but to make you think it out for yourself.

— Elbert Hubbard

8

ABUNDANT PROTEIN
WITHOUT MEAT

You do not have to eat expensive meat in order to give your body the protein it needs. Having many trips around the world and thirteen expeditions into primitive parts of the world, I have found thousands of men and women who were fantastic physical specimens, who never touched meat.

Several years ago while doing nutritional research in Guatemala I saw the greatest demonstration of group endurance and physical strength that I ever witnessed in my life. It was done by men and women of all ages, as well as children. And these people did not eat one mouthful of meat during this grueling test of strength and endurance.

Here is how it happened. I was at the great market place in Guatemala City where I saw men with 125 pounds of lumber strapped on their backs. The women carried 80 pounds and the children carried lesser amounts. They were taking this finished lumber high into their village in the mountains.

AN ARDUOUS JOURNEY WITHOUT MEAT

I went along with these people and observed their diet during the trip. They had no meat of any kind. Here's what their diet consisted of: raw vegetables, fruit, goat's cheese, beans, sunflower seeds, eggs, pumpkin seeds, and whole cornmeal bread.

Just think of it! Men with 125 pounds of lumber strapped on their backs, climbing mountains. An to top it off, they were gay and happy as they climbed. At the end of the day, the men, women and children would sing and dance with no apparent loss of energy, strength and vitality. To me this was a great demonstration that people can endure the greatest physical strains and live happily and healthily on a vegetarian diet.

HEALTH AND VITALITY IN AFRICA'S ATLAS MOUNTAINS

Across the Atlantic Ocean in the Atlas Mountains of northwest Africa, I also found vegetarians of similar strength and stamina. The people of this region live on a vegetarian diet and maintain beautiful bodies, with great endurance and energy. Hiking with great loads on their backs does not seem to strain them. After a strenuous day of hard physical labor, they appear in village squares and dance the native dances with tremendous vigor. Their diet consists of fruits, vegetables, olive oil, chick-peas (garbanzos), eggs, brown rice, almonds, goat's cheese, various beans and whole grain breads and dates.

ARAB VEGETARIANS IN THE SAHARA DESERT

In my nutritional research in Africa's great Sahara Desert I found some of the greatest specimens of manhood and womanhood. The men here are considered the greatest horsemen in the world. They are also splendid acrobats, and noted for their skilled feats of strength, agility and balance. I have seen one of these acrobats support five large men standing on his shoulders. The diet is a most simple vegetarian diet: largely dates, dried figs, raisins, cheese and brown rice.

INDIA PRODUCES MANY STRONG PEOPLE ON A VEGETARIAN DIET

Many people have the preconceived idea that all the inhabitants of India are victims of malnutrition. This is far from the truth. In parts of India, powerful men and women are products of a vegetarian diet.

Mahatma Gandhi, one of the greatest men of our time, was a vegetarian. I had the extreme honor of this man's friendship, and have hiked miles with him over rough, dusty, hot, treacherous roads in India. Although of small physical stature, in endurance and stamina he was a superman.

Health and cheerfulness make beauty.

—Cervantes

In my nutritional researches in India I found yogis (strict vegetarians) who were physical marvels. India has produced extraordinarily great athletes, some over six feet tall, on an exclusively vegetarian diet. I had the pleasure of meeting the great wrestler, Gama, who during his prime could defeat any man in the world. He was a strict vegetarian.

175 YEARS OF VEGETARIANISM IN ENGLAND

In England there are thousands of vegetarians. I have had the pleasure of meeting great musicians, writers, physicians, artists and many others in all walks of life who are strict vegetarians. There are Vegetarian Societies in England that have been in continuous existence for over 175 years.

The great writer, George Bernard Shaw, was my personal friend and one of the great vegetarians of all time. He lived into his nineties with a sharp, clear, intelligent mind. He met his death falling out of an apple tree he was pruning. But for this accident, I believe Mr. Shaw would still be living a vigorous life at well over 100 years of age.

GREAT VEGETARIANS OF THE PAST

Some of the most brillant and intelligent minds throughout history have been nurtured on a vegetarian diet. Among these are some of the world's greatest philosophers including Pythagoras, Plato, Plutarch, Diogenes, and St. Chrysostum. The genius Leonardo da Vinci was a vegetarian. So were Benjamin Franklin, John Wesley, Emanuel Swedenborg, Henry David Thoreau, Francois Voltaire, John Howard, Sir Richard Philips, Percy Blysse Shelley, William Wordsworth, Milton Pope, and Professor Arnold Ehret.

One of the best known vegetarians of our time is Dr. John Harvey Kellogg, founder and director of the great Battle Creek Sanitarium in Battle Creek, Michigan, who retired at 96 years of age. The Seventh Day Adventist Church was founded by a vegetarian, Ellen G. White.

Space does not permit me to name other greats who have been vegetarians throughout the ages.

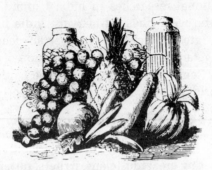

FRUITARIANS—A TYPE OF VEGETARIANISM

In my travels over the world I have met vegetarians who are really what we would call fruitarians, or grugivorous, as they live exclusively on fruits. A current example is the noted comedian, Dick Gregory, who has just written a best seller entitled, *Dick Gregory's Natural Diet for Folks Who Eat: Cookin' with Mother Nature*. Excessively overweight before he started his fruitarian diet, Gregory has lost almost 200 pounds.

Fruitarians claim that man was intended to eat only fruit, citing as their premise Genesis 1:29 (Revised Standard Version):

"And God said, 'Behold, I have given you every plant yielding seed which is upon the face of the earth, and every tree with seed in its fruit; you shall have them for food."

The King James Version translates the same verse in these words: "And God said, Behold I have given you every herb bearing seed, which is upon the face of all the earth, and every tree, in the which is the fruit of a tree yielding seed; to you it shall be for *meat*."

Thus the story of creation in the Bible indicates that fruit is the food human beings are intended to eat, and that the word "meat" itself in this context means fruit rather than animal flesh.

As a matter of fact, the physical makeup of the human body supports this interpretation. The human physiology has more in common with the frugivorous than the carnivorous, or flesh-eating, members of the animal kingdom.

First of all, flesh-eating animals have a very short intestinal tract. This is necessary because of the highly putrefactive character of the food they eat. Human beings, on the other hand, have very long intestinal tracts, as do other members of the animal kingdom who subsist on a vegetarian diet. This would indicate that Mother Nature never intended a flesh diet for humans. We just don't have the guts for it, so to speak. And when you consider (as we shall do later) the problems of elimination suffered by meat-eating (in the non-Biblical sense of flesh) humans, the original blueprint seems to be vegetarian.

Secondly, carnivorous animals are provided with special teeth or fangs to seize their prey and tear off the flesh, as well as crack the bones. Human beings, however, in common with apes and chimpanzees and other herbivorous (vegetarian) animals, lack such dental equipment. Apes, for example, could never manage to eat the carcasses of large animals—nor could humans until they invented knives! An examination of human teeth indicates that they are better suited to masticate pulpy fruits, succulent stems and leaves, rather than flesh.

Finally, the digestive juices of human beings indicate that Mother Nature did not intend her human children to be carnivorous. The digestion of flesh and bone requires large amounts of hydrochloric acid, which is supplied in concentrated form in the digestive tracts of carnivorous animals. Humans do not have this natural capacity.

Accepting such physical evidence and the word of scripture, fruitarians interpret these literally to apply to a diet exclusively of fruit, direct from plants and trees—in a natural state, fully "cooked" by Mother Nature's outdoor oven of sun, light, air and moisture. Some go a step further and add nuts to the diet.

VEGANS—ANOTHER TYPE OF VEGETARIAN

I have also met vegetarians who extend this interpretation to mean the inclusion of vegetables, nuts, grains and seeds, along with fruits. They are known as "vegans".

Vegans reject milk, cheese, eggs, and all foods coming from animals. In addition to health considerations in connection

13

with diet, veganism is based on the moral conviction that nothing which has to be killed should be eaten.

LACTO-VEGETARIANS—THE MOST POPULAR TYPE

The most successful vegetarians I have met over the world are the lacto-vegetarians. In fact, this is what most people mean when they refer to vegetarianism. It is the type of vegetarianism practiced by the famous vegetarians whom I named previously, including Mahatma Gandhi.

Lacto-vegetarianism—to which I shall refer to hereafter simply as "vegetarianism"—consists of eating plant substances such as fruits, vegetables, whole grains and cereals, nuts and seeds, along with milk, natural milk products, fertile eggs and honey. This is a nutritionally well balanced diet, easily and naturally assimilated by the human body.

VEGETARIANS EXCEL AS ATHLETES

Having been an athlete for more than 60 years, taking part in many different types of athletic sports such as swimming, tennis, high mountain climbing, long distance running, volleyball, bicycling and wrestling, I have met many vegetarians who are outstanding athletes. Many of these were competitors in the Olympic Games. Murray Rose, for example, who won five gold medals for his swimming feats in the Olympics, has been a vegetarian since infancy.

It has been erroneously believed that vegetarians could not compete with flesh-eaters in athletic events. Recent experiments show this to be absolutely false.

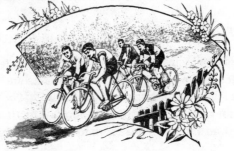

Five years ago, while I was doing research on the athletic abilities of vegetarians vs. meat-eaters, I was a spectator at the great walk from Berlin to Vienna, a distance of 361 miles. Vegetarians were so far ahead of the flesh-eaters that the flesh-eaters were really not "in it" at all.

At another walking match in Germany, 13 vegetarians and 26 flesh-eaters entered the 40-mile walking contest. The first two to reach the finish line were vegetarians. In other contest, I saw vegetarians win races of 100 miles over flesh-eaters.

Several years ago I was a spectator at the race from Colorado Springs to the top of Pikes Peak. Several hundred athletes took part in this great endurance test—and the first three men to reach the top were vegetarians.

The winner of this endurance race was 56 years of age, running against men who could have been his sons. When I asked him why he was a vegetarian, he replied, "I personally eat no animal food because, like the Buddhists, I do not consider it right to take what I cannot give—life; because I do not think it is right to cause pain to the lower orders of creation because eating meat excites, stimulates and increases the vitality of the animal nature; and further, I partake of no meat because even in the healthiest cattle, pork and sheep there is more or less waste matter, dead substance in the muscles and the blood, not removed by the circulation—and I insist it's putrefactive matter, this dead broken-down tissue in meat and blood and liver of slain beasts, not fit to eat."

DEGENERATIVE DISEASES IN AN AFFLUENT SOCIETY

Those who eat fruit, vegetables, whole grains, seeds, nuts, eggs and dairy products get their nourishment in all its purity from the original source—while flesh-eaters get all this second-hand, re-chewing and re-digesting that which has already once been assimilated.

During the past 30-odd years, we Americans have become an affluent society, and more people can afford to eat meat several times a day (even at rising prices). In fact, Americans consume more meat than any other nation in the world. Meat three times

15

a day is not a rare occurence ... ham or bacon with eggs for breakfast; hamburgers, hot dogs or luncheon meat for lunch; with steak, chops or roast as the main dish of the typical American dinner.

If you stop and look around you, you can see the sad results of eating large amounts of meat. You will see young people becoming prematurely old at 25 and 35 years of age, many with cholesterol buildup and hardening of the arteries. The clogging of the arteries by cholesterol from animal fats, called arteriosclerosis, is considered a major signpost of the aging process—i.e., a degenerative process, not due to the number of years one has lived but to how one has lived them. The prevalence of arteriosclerosis at an early calendar age in Americans was shockingly discovered during the Korean war, when examination of the bodies of young soldiers killed in battle revealed that 77% of the Americans (average age 22) already had arteriosclerosis. In contrast, among the Koreans and other Orientals who had died on the same battlefield under the same conditions, there was only 11% incidence of this disease. As is well known, the Oriental diet is low in animal fats.

Take five average Americans today, put them together in a living room and start talking about physical ailments. You will hear about varicose veins, swollen ankles, arthritis, ulcers, gallstones, prostate gland trouble, hemorrhoids, liver trouble, female trouble, skin trouble, nervousness, overweight, underweight, bad feet, headaches, shortness of breath, insomnia, lack of energy, fatigue, and many other ailments.

As meat eating has increased during the past years in the USA, the kidney ailment known as Bright's Disease has increased 65%; heart trouble, 300%; epilepsy, 450%; and insanity 400%. While we have the reputation of raising the so-called "best" cattle, all forms of human degenerative diseases are on the increase. Doesn't this look suspicious?

Americans' main food is meat, and it also takes the highest amount of the food budget. And are we actually getting toxins such as uric acid and cholesterol. These are difficult enough for the human body to handle. But commercially raised animals today, especially cattle and poultry, are usually penned up so they do not get normal exercise, and are given chemical additives in their food (and sometimes injections) to accelerate growth and add weight. Then, after they are butchered, more chemicals are added as preservatives. The meat is already unhealthy before it comes to market. No wonder meat-eating Americans are prey to degenerative diseases!

ANIMAL PROTEINS AND FATS
CONNECTED WITH CANCER

Cancer of the large intestine (colon-rectal) is the most common major cancer in the USA, and is second only to lung cancer in the number of cancer deaths, according to recent reports in the WALL STREET JOURNAL and the LOS ANGELES TIMES. Highest incidence of such bowel cancer is found in beef-producing, beef-eating countries—the USA, Scotland and Denmark (the three countries with the highest death rate from this cause), Argentina, Uruguay, New Zealand, Canada and Ireland.

A diet survey by the U.S. Department of Agriculture revealed that the 28-year-old male American (taken as the average) consumes almost 90% more protein, primarily meat, than recommended by official national standards.

Dr. Willard Visek, professor of animal science at Cornell University, points out that this high intake of animal protein results—through computer-like reactions of body chemistry——in higher concentrations of toxic ammonia in the large intestine. Ammonia has a number of characteristics of a chemical carcinogen (a compound which induces cancer formation). It destroys cells; alters nucleic acid (DNA and RNA) synthesis; alters growth of transplantable tumors in animals; harms noncancerous cells more than cancerous cells; and increases virus infections.

Dr. Ernest L. Wynder, president of the American Health Foundation and a long-time cancer researcher, notes that 45% of the American diet consists of fats, chiefly animal which produce abnormal chemical reactions in the large intestine.

Reporting on a recent study of the National Cancer Institute in Hawaii, Dr. William Haenszel and Dr. John Berg said that immigrants from Japan—where bowel cancer rate is low—have developed a high incidence of colon-rectal cancer after switching from the traditional Japanese diet of vegetables and fish to the meat-heavy, fat-heavy American diet.

 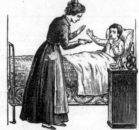

OUR MALNOURISHED YOUTH

Americans, especially young Americans, are snack eaters——and the more they snack, the more disease increases. Millions of hot dogs are consumed daily, millions of pounds of greasy fried chicken and cremated hamburgers—which is helping to destroy the health of our nation.

I have made very careful research among teenagers, and found that many of them suffer from malnutrition because they are not eating, and are not conditioned to eat, natural foods such as fruits and vegetables. They eat processed hydrogenized salted peanut butter, empty calorie processed cereals, and consume enormous quantities of candy, cake, pie, commercial ice cream—made from refined white flour and sugar—and other foodless foods.

I personally believe that the drug habit can be closely associated with malnutrition. At high school and college sports events, I am amazed at the amount of "junk" (garbage) food and drink that are consumed by the young people—candy bars, cola drinks, over-salted popcorn, doughnuts, cupcakes, as well as hot dogs, hamburgers, fried chicken, pizza pie, ice cream, malts and French fries.

Many young people never get an adequate amount of first-class proteins—and as their energy dips, they turn to stimulants such as alcohol, tobacco and drugs. You can't expect to build a healthy body with potato chips, salted peanuts, cookies, and food made with refined white flour and refined white sugar.

The modern process of robbing the nourishment from natural foods embalming them for shelf-life and profit completely thwarts Nature's inviolable program. Bread, for example, can no longer be called the "staff of life". The natural, life-giving vitamins, minerals and nutrients of the wheat have been refined out of bleached flour—leaving merely empty calories quickly converted into energy, but with no elements for body building and repairing.

If we're going to preserve the health of our nation, we must teach the young people the value of natural foods!

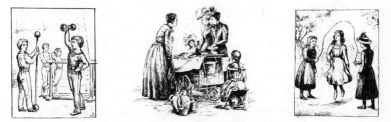

YOUNG PEOPLE ARE AWAKENING
TO THE IMPORTANCE OF GOOD NUTRITION

As my lecture work carries me all over the world, I do see a ray of hope shining brightly for the young people. Many of them are beginning to realize that the vegetarian diet is the most wholesome of all diets. Some of our best young people are changing their ancestral eating habits. Because of their deep reverence for all living creatures, they are going vegetarian.

Young people are opening natural health food restaurants from one end of the country to another, selling exclusively vegetarian foods. I have just finished a nationwide lecture tour, and in city after city I found young people conducting successful vegetarian restaurants.

Right here in Hawaii, where I now make my home, are some of the finest vegetarian restaurants in the world, most of them operated by young people. Not only are young people and others turning to vegetarianism because of their deep reverence

19

for all living creatures. They are also aware of the current risky practices in raising poultry and livestock with the use of antibiotics and stilbestrol in animal feed, the use of tranquilizers, and the spraying of animal feed with insecticides. We must concede that meat, unless you can get it from organic sources, does have its quota of dangers.

A MEATLESS DIET MUST AVOID PROTEIN DEFICIENCY

I definitely believe that it is possible to have health, strength, endurance and vigor on a purely vegetarian diet, but it is not easy and that is the reason I am writing this book. One should not undertake the vegetarian diet in a haphazard manner. It is true that many famous people have lived their lives well without meat. However, bear in mind that when these men and women lived, vegetables, fruits, nuts, grains and dairy products still had all the nutrients nature intended them to have.

Today, because of poor farming practices and the use of chemical fertilizers, our soils have become depleted. Every year the nutrition that is delivered, in ratio to the products grown, becomes less and less.

The U.S. Department of Agriculture, when it pats itself on the back for its great food production, bases its yearly statistics not on nutrients but on the yield per acre. The protein content of wheat, oats, barley, millet, soy beans, dried legumes and corn grown in the United States is steadily declining, even as the bushel yield of grain per acre is increasing.

On research, I have found that the protein content of all grains is declining on an average of 1% per year. That is the reasons it's so important, when going on a vegetarian diet, that you eat food produced on organic soil. Of course, the best way to get organically grown foods is to grow them yourself. A small area in your backyard can produce vegetables and salad greens for your needs. Tomatoes can be grown in pots in an apartment, where window boxes and inside planters can make a real garden. Sprouts, almost 100% protein, can be grown in a glass jar.

Remember, every one of the billions of cells of your body—a quadrillion of them—NEED PROTEIN DAILY. It is deep down in the fantastically intricate mechanism of each of these cells that good health begins or fails to begin, depending upon the quality of the protein and the nutrients with which we provide these cells.

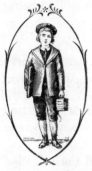

HUMAN INDIVIDUALITY

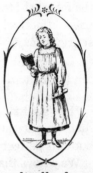

Science has established that cells differ so radically from organ to organ, and the bodies composed of those cells and organs differ so drastically from individual to individual, that the unique nutritional requirements of each human being are more distinct than his fingertips—and far more complex. Science knows, furthermore, that the shapes, sizes, circulatory supply lines and metabolic performances (food-burning and nutrient conversion capabilities) of our various organs differ greatly from person to person.

What does this biological fact of life tell us? Loud and clear it says that there is no such statistical abstraction as "the average man and woman". Each person is biologically an individual and—in ways that can spell the difference between good health and something that is too often far less—is distinct from other bodies in terms of food requirements.

Because this is so, the odds are overwhelming that in our nutritionally backward, food-industry, homogenized society, even the best fed among us are like corn trying to grow in a not too fertile, nutrient-starved soil. At the cellular level, where it really counts, we are usually not getting anything like optimal nutrition. Therefore, it is absolutely essential that the approximately 40 vitamins, minerals and amino acids (protein) every

21

human body requires daily to enjoy radiant health, be supplied in combination and work together as a unit.

When a single nutrient seems to be acting by itself—for example, if B-1 appears to cure beriberi or ascorbic acid eliminates scurvy—that is not what is really happening. These vitamins by themselves could not do their work at all were it not for the fact that other necessary nutrients are present and are being used effectively. To bring a victim of beriberi, pellagra or scurvy back to health, full nutrition is essential.

300,000 RETARDANTS BORN EACH YEAR IN THE U.S.

Here's what we must face. In living on a meat or vegetarian diet, we must supply the body with all the nutrients to keep the body in perfect working order.

We know that a diet made up exclusively of the so-called "fun foods" of adolescents (cola drinks, potato chips, refined white flour and white sugar products, fried potatoes, candy bars and all calory-laden sweets) cause malnutrition of the brain and markedly erodes brain cells, paving the way for later, mental illness. Yet youngsters and parents receive most of their food information from TV advertising, and are not getting in the public schools the health-maintenance advice they should be getting.

We know that the body stands stress—but with plenty of pantothenic acid, an essential B-complex nutrient. We know that Vitamin B-6 (pyridoxine) which, because of today's trash diets, is often a weak link in the nutritional chain, is vital in helping psychotic children.

We know that most people suffering from pernicious-anemia, who lack Vitamin B-12, have characteristic mood depression; and so have people who lack B-1 and B-2 biotin (B-complex growth vitamin) and folic acid (folic acid is commonly deficient among elderly psychotic people). The absence of one or more of these essential substances can also cause hallucinations, severe agitation, maniac behavior, inability to concentrate, groundless panic, memory loss, sensitivity to noise, lassitude, and withdrawal states.

To supply the brain with its food requirements, including Vitamins B-1, B-2, B-3, B-6, B-12 and C, biotin, folic acid, iodine, magnesium, calcium and the amino acids (protein), we must have a complete eating program which includes every nutrient the human body needs to maintain health.

We know certain food deficiencies produce cataracts in animals. We nutritionists believe that good nutrition can prevent them in humans.

HOW TO SOLVE YOUR NUTRITIONAL PROBLEMS

Every person who desires radiant health, whether he includes or excludes meat, should have a basic knowledge of how food (initially a part of our internal environment) determines proper balances in the body's eternal ecology.

It is simple to eat foods as close to nature as possible. A diet composed of a plentiful supply of raw fruit and vegetables and properly cooked vegetables, natural cheeses, eggs, nuts, seeds and whole grains, would afford more enjoyment and a much superior state of health, with a far longer life expectancy. In eating a diet of this kind, all the essential nutrients are supplied to the body; and a computer is not required in the kitchen to formulate a good, wholesome, healthy diet.

Personally, I believe that which is not simple and easy to understand is confusing. Therefore, keep this in mind when purchasing food. Do as much of your shopping as possible in the health food stores. These people are in the business of supplying super-nutrition, they have the organic foods, they have the unprocessed foods, they have the unsprayed foods, and they can supply you with the food supplements that you need to round out a program of balanced nutrition. Many health food stores have available the organic fruits and vegetables.

California is the most advanced state in supplying organic foods, and the other states of the union could really learn a lesson in how to raise the standard of health by following the advances that have been made by the health food advocates of California.

HOW MUCH PROTEIN DOES THE BODY NEED?

For over sixty years as a biochemist and nutritionist, I have been researching on the amount of protein each human should have daily, and I have come to the conclusion that it is anywhere from 50 to 75 grams, depending on your size and your physical activity. Naturally, a husky man is going to require more protein than a small child, but no one from a teenager on should have less than 50 grams each day. EXCEPTIONS—on fasting day, when you drink distilled water only. I faithfully fast one 24-hour period weekly which helps keep my body toxin free. Read "The Miracle of Fasting," for ordering, see back cover.

Protein, as we know, is found in meat, but protein is also in fish, fowl, cheese, milk products, eggs, nuts, seeds, whole grains and beans. As I have stated, the quadrillion cells of your body are made of protein.

How you look today, how you feel today, the energy you have, your disposition, all depend on a balanced nutrition within the body chemistry. Looking and feeling your best is important to you, so let's get down to facts about protein.

The most important fact for you to remember is that your skin, your nails, and your hair all have one great essential ingredient, and that's protein. Protein is your number one food.

There are many places where protein starvation will show up in your body. One is your skin tone. Look around you and observe the skin condition of the average human. It is either flabby or pudgy, with puffiness under the eyes and skin drooping over the eyelids.

Not only is protein deficiency evident in the skin, but protein deficiency shows up in the tone of the flesh or muscles of the body. In other words, an adequate amount of protein helps build healthy skin tone and muscle tone.

Every man is the builder of a temple called his body . . . We are all sculptors and painters, and our material is our own flesh and blood and bones. Any nobleness begins at once to refine a man's features, any meanness or sensuality to imbrute them.

— Henry David Thoreau

24

PROTEIN-HUNGRY HAIR

Your hair is another place where protein deficiency is going to show up, because if your body needs that protein to maintain its general health, it really isn't going to care whether your hair is looking healthy with a good sheen—but you care!

As you look around, you'll see that some hair is dry and looks like straw while other hair is oily and greasy and unmanagable. If your hair is luxuriant, it's a good barometer to tell you that you're getting an adequate amount of protein.

One of the best protein sources for the health of your hair and your body in general is found in fertile eggs. The egg is a storehouse of nutritional treasures. It is not only a fine source of protein, but the egg also contains two of the most important B vitamins for the hair and body—choline and inositol, part of the B-complex.

Many people have been frightened away from eating eggs with scare literature stating that the cholesterol in eggs can kill you. I will admit there is cholesterol in eggs, but eggs also contain the anti-cholesterol agent, lecithin. During my many years as a nutritionist, I have found that three or four eggs can be used by an adult every week and a growing child can eat as many as two eggs daily, because the growing body uses more protein.

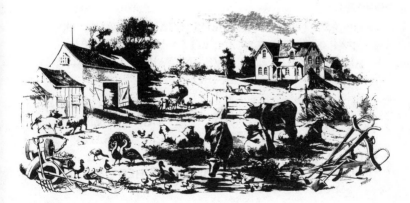

SPROUTS
A TREMENDOUS SOURCE
OF VEGETABLE PROTEIN

Sprouts are an important food for vegetarians. Most of the vegetables purchased at the supermarket are not providing the nutrients which you should have. If you are on a vegetarian diet, and especially if you are a vegan and not consuming dairy products or eggs, this could be disastrous. By all means, whether you're on a meat diet or a vegetarian diet, get your vegetables, nuts, grains, seeds and beans from organic sources. Best of all, have a home organic garden. If that is not possible, then you can raise your own sprouts anywhere. Alfalfa and other sprouts can be your lifeline to radiant health on a vegetarian diet—and just think of it, they can be grown anywhere! Ask at your health food store for instructions.

Many grains and seeds contain beneficial nutrients when they are sprouted because they undergo organic changes which multiply their vitamin, mineral, enzyme and protein content. I have found in my long experience as a nutritionist that sprouted grains and legumes provide enough first quality proteins to be classed as absolutely complete. They pass the test which is used to determine the completeness of a food; they sustain life all through the reproductive cycle for several generations.

LEARN TO SPROUT SEEDS, BEANS, GRAINS TO
REAP MORE PROTEIN, VITAMINS, MINERALS,
AMINO ACIDS AND LIVE ENZYMES COMPARED
TO THEIR DRY STATE.

ALFALFA SEEDS   GARBANZO BEANS
LENTILS   MUNG BEANS
NAVY BEANS   PINTO BEANS
SOY BEANS
WHEAT, TRITICALE WHEAT, And OTHER GRAINS.

Example to show you the great difference — The soybean in the dry stage has little Vitamin C — but after sprouting for 3 days, the Vitamin C count jumps up equal to six glasses of fresh orange juice per ½ cup of sprouts.

Alfalfa seed sprouts are a super food for vegetarians and can substitute for supermarket vegetables when it's impossible to get organic ones. Remember to use only untreated seeds for sprouting. Many commercial seeds are treated with fungicides like mercury, which are deadly.

YOU MUST HAVE ALL THE AMINO ACIDS

When planning a vegetarian diet, be sure that you get all of the amino acids. It's the amino acids which become the protein of your body. Eggs and dairy products are complete proteins, which means they contain all the essential amino acids in the correct proportions.

All but eight of the known amino acids can be synchronized by your body from other sources. They are, therefore, not called essential. The eight which you must include in your diet because the body cannot make them, are: leucine, methionine, phenylanine, valine, lysine, isoleucine, threonine and trytophan.

The three great building blocks of protein are lysine, methionine and cystine. The soy bean is the most perfect of all the vegetarian foods and should be used several times a week.

VEGETARIAN FOODS THAT ARE RICH IN AMINO ACIDS

When avocados, seeds and nuts are eaten with raw, green leafy vegetables, they provide a complete amino acid pattern that is well utilized by the body. Raw and roasted peanuts are a wonderful source of vegetable amino acids. A sandwich made of 100% whole wheat (toast all bread), with natural peanut butter (contains no salt, sugar or preservatives) from the health food store, lettuce, tomato, sunflower seeds and sliced raw mushrooms supplies practically all of your amino acids.

Health and good humor are to the body what sunshine is to vegetation.

—Massillon

I find that a salad made of lettuce, tomatoes, cucumbers, cabbage, celery, beets, avocado, hard boiled egg, cheese and sunflower seeds again supplies most of the amino acids. A sandwich made of whole grain bread, alfalfa sprouts, lettuce, tomato, raw mushrooms, natural cheddar cheese and health mayonnaise gives practically all of the aminos.

A peanut butter sandwich (add sesame seeds to peanut butter), watercress, alfalfa sprouts, grated carrots, and 2 hard boiled egg gives you a biologically complete lunch with most of the amino acids. Along with the sandwich, you could munch a variety of raw nuts. Cashew nuts rate high in lysine; sesame and sunflower seeds are excellent sources of methionine.

Millet is a good high protein cereal which every vegetarian should include in his diet. So are buckwheat groats, whole unpearled barley, natural whole grain brown rice, and soy beans, which come closest of all the plant foods to being a complete protein.

B-12 SUPPLEMENT ESSENTIAL IN VEGETARIAN DIET

The major deficiency which must be guarded against in a vegetarian diet is Vitamin B-12, an essential in the B-complex and considered crucial in preventing anemia. As previously stated, there is no known practical plant source that supplies an adequate amount of Vitamin B-12. Kelp, as noted, is the best plant source. Comfrey leaves have a small amount of B-12. Yeast, wheat germ and soy beans also have traces.

Eggs and milk products contain some Vitamin B-12. But none of the components of a vegetarian diet contain enough.

Let me warn you that folic acid (another member of the B-complex vitamins), which is plentiful in green vegetables, can make the blood analysis often appear normal—and thus prevent the detection of a Vitamin B-12 deficiency before nerve damage occurs.

To be nutritionally safe, it would certainly be wise for everyone on a vegetarian diet, and especially vegans, to include a daily B supplement that is rich in B-12—and thus avoid the possibility of a nervous condition which may not show its symptoms for ten years. B-12 is made from molds. It is not synthetic nor of animal origin when you get it as a supplement.

RAW FRESH WHEAT GERM
ALSO ESSENTIAL IN A VEGETARIAN DIET

As a nutritionist and biochemist, I have a high regard for the exceptional nutritional value of raw wheat germ, which contains one of the most precious of all vitamins—Vitamin E. It has been called the "wonder food" as it is almost a complete food in itself. It is a rich source of high quality protein and contains Vitamin B complex, iron, phosporus, Vitamin E and many other powerful nutritive elements not found in abundance in other foods.

In my athletic career, I was constantly searching for a wonder food to give me that extra vitality, endurance and strength to be a winner. As stated in this book, I have been an active athlete all my life, with the exception of a two-year period between the ages of 16 and 18 when I was recovering from tuberculosis in a Swiss sanitorium. It was during this miraculous change from a sick body to a vital, healthy body that I dedicated my life as a young boy to help others to health as I had been helped by these wonderful Swiss doctors who believed in working with Nature and her helpers—sunshine, fresh air, natural foods, and pure, distilled water.

HOW I DISCOVERED
THE NUTRITIONAL VALUE OF RAW WHEAT GERM

In the early 1920's I was on a research project in Texas. Here's how I made my discovery of the nutritional power of raw wheat germ. Our nutritional group was studying animals, both male and female, who could no longer reproduce themselves and were turned loose in a large fenced field. The worn-out male bulls and the cows had absolutely no interest in each other. Their sexual powers seemed to have ceased to exist. The group made many test feedings to see if we could revive the reproductive forces in these animals. But time after time we failed.

Near the feeding pens of these animals was a large flour mill.

29

One day while I was visiting this mill, I saw wagons being loaded with raw natural wheat germ which had been extracted from the wheat in the mill. I asked one of the men driving one of the large wagons what he was going to do with the raw wheat germ, and he said, "I'm taking it to a dump to be thrown away."

I said to the man, "Would you drive the wagon into the feeding pen where those animals are?" He replied that it would be indeed a pleasure since it would save him a five-mile trip to the dump.

So I had five wagon loads of raw wheat germ dumped into the feeding pens where the experiment with the depleted animals was going on. All of the animals, both male and female, disregarded the other foods and made a dash to consume as much of the raw wheat germ as they could eat.

In 72 hours of this feeding on raw wheat germ, a miracle seemed to happen in the feeding pens. The male and the female animals were again becoming interested in each other sexually. In about three weeks of this kind of feeding, these animals took on an entirely different appearance. Their eyes became bright, their hides became silky and shining, and instead of the lethargy that had previously characterized these animals, they were acting like young animals.

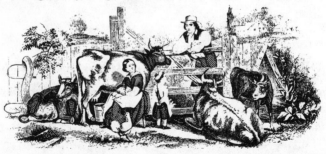

I then started feeding raw wheat germ and wheat germ oil to athletes. Again, this wonder food performed a miracle on these athletes. The sprinters specializing in the 100-yard and the 200-yard dash reduced their time in these events by from 1 to 5 seconds. This demonstrated to me not only the value of wheat germ, but also the value of exercise related to good nutrition.

I then took a group of athletes, fed them raw natural wheat germ and trained them with the specific objective of increasing their endurance. I used cross-country runners covering 5 to 10 miles over hilly country. These athletes on this raw wheat germ diet improved steadily for three months.

I found to my surprise that men training hard over a period of three or four months eating the ordinary diet would, as we say in the vernacular of athletes, "go stale". Their energy, endurance and athletic ability would go into a slump. When I fed these athletes raw wheat germ, they lost this staleness, or dip in their athletic ability, and seemed to gain more power in their athletic performance.

One of the dishes I fed these athletes was plain yogurt, raw wheat germ and raw honey. With this added to a good health diet, the athletes started breaking many records.

I have not only used raw wheat germ on athletes, but also on weak children, weak teenagers and weak adults, and I have found this vegetarian dish of yogurt, raw wheat germ and honey a nutritional powerhouse.

So it is my conviction that all vegetarians should use raw wheat germ in their diet daily.

If you attend any great athletic event, such as the Olympics, you will find that wheat germ and wheat germ oil is used quite extensively by the competing athletes.

COMBINE GOOD NUTRITION WITH EXERCISE

I believe it is very necessary for every athlete, if he wants to be a champion in his event, to depend not only on his native strength, endurance and athletic training, but to look to good nutrition as an aid in achieving more proficiency.

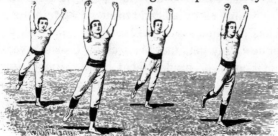

This book is not written for athletes alone since I believe everyone should have an exercise program, regardless of his calendar years, if the exercise is nothing more than a two mile brisk walk. More pleasure and enjoyment can be derived from walking, or any other physical exercise, if a plan of good nutrition is followed, including the use of raw wheat germ.

I believe there is in raw wheat germ and wheat germ oil an X-factor which has not been isolated, since it has been my experience with athletes and others who are physically active that it does increase pep and endurance.

BREWER'S YEAST AS A VEGETABLE PROTEIN - PLUS

Brewer's yeast is an almost incredibly nutritive food. It contains 50% high quality complete protein—and is also a gold mine of rare vitamins and minerals that help prevent degenerative diseases . . . plus abundant nucleic acids that have been found effective in rejuvenation.

I believe that everyone on a vegetation diet should use at least a tablespoonful of Brewer's yeast daily. It can be placed in blender drinks, vegetarian loaves, vegetarian patties or burgers or sprinkled over vegetables, cereals, etc. It can be mixed with salad dressings, or can simply be taken in juice.

Brewer's yeast, with its 50% protein, contains practically all of the known amino acid building blocks needed for the construction of tissue and the maintenance of body functions. It also contains practically all of the important B-complex vitamins so valuable to super-health and vitality.

Not only does Brewer's yeast contain proteins, vitamins and minerals, but it is rich in nucleic acid found within the nuclei of all living cells, which is now known to contain the very blueprints by which all organs and tissues maintain the proper number of healthy functioning cells.

I have found in my personal research on Brewer's yeast that this element known as nucleic acid has an almost uncanny ability to help to turn back the clock, to retard the onset of premature aging; in effect, to recharge the battery of your worn-out cells, thus giving them a renewed capacity to create the mysterious conditions that give you the look and feel of youth.

When you look at the skin on the back of an aged hand, what deficiency has caused the hand to become spotted, brittle, shiny and wrinkled? The answer is that the nucleic acids of the cells have lost the ability to reproduce clearly all the blueprints they contain, which govern the formation of new cells, to replace those that have deteriorated with the passage of time.

In my nutritional investigations I have found great improvement in aging bodies with the use of Brewer's yeast, which is about 15% nucleic acid. I have found that the daily use of Brewer's yeast helps increase the energy and the feeling of wellbeing. I have found that people who use Brewer's yeast daily find alteration in skin aspect towards a healthier, rosier looking skin and simultaneously an apparent smoothing of the skin of the face.

I find that people who use Brewer's yeast daily increase in skin tightness and in the moistures of the skin as well. Other areas that show improvment are the elbows and other joints, where the roughness of the skin diminishes. The skin of the back of the hand has improved in smoothness in many people within five or six months.

The important trace mineral—zinc—is also plentiful in Brewer's yeast, as well as in nuts and raw wheat germ.

I feel that the daily use of Brewer's yeast will help you feel younger, look younger and possess better resistance to the illnesses that come increasingly as we live longer. You couldn't do better than to include in your diet a tablespoonful of Brewer's yeast every single day of your life.

BUCKWHEAT LEADS ALL GRAINS IN PROTEIN

So many people who feel that meat is expensive would like to try a vegetarian diet, eating more vegetables and grains, but they just don't like soybeans which is one of the foods in the vegetable kingdom highest in protein. They know they need protein . . . so where else can they go to get their protein in large quantities except soybeans? The answer is buckwheat.

Very few people know that buckwheat is an excellent source of high quality protein and that it tastes good. In the hands of a good cook, it can be a delicious and nutritious food. Buckwheat is an inexpensive and nutritious main or side dish. It is very low in calories for a food with starch content. Buckwheat has fewer calories than wheat, barley, rye or brown rice. Buckwheat is a superior source of protein and is high in manganese, iron, magnesium, thiamine, and riboflavin. It has almost all the food values of a thick, juicy beef steak and can appreciably lower anyone's food budget.

One of the reasons buckwheat is so inexpensive is that it is easily grown. It requires only a small amount of fertilizer and is strong and hearty, being almost immune to disease. It has a great natural resistance to insects and is rarely sprayed with herbicides, weed killers or pesticides. Buckwheat has super-vitality and grows so swiftly that it smothers any weeds growing around it. It is used as a "weed smother crop" to kill out fields infested with crabgrass. It grows very rapidly and in two months is ready for harvesting. A good yield is about twenty bushels per acre.

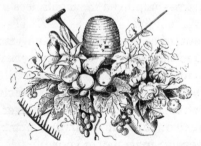

Farmers have been using buckwheat to produce a honey crop. Buckwheat honey has an exceptional flavor and is dark and rich. It is in special demand and commands high prices. Bees can take 160 pounds of honey from one acre of buckwheat under good growing conditions in a single season, although nectar flows only during the morning.

When we analyze buckwheat we find it contains between 12% and 16% protein. Just think of it! There is more protein in buckwheat than whole grain wheat and even in cooked soybeans, and it comes closer to animal protein than any other grain crop. Buckwheat protein has between 7% and 9% of the amino acid lysine which is even more than high-lysine corn.

Both rye and wheat are deficient in lysine which makes their protein lowgrade. But protein in buckwheat flour, without any amino acid additions, has the same nutritive quality as proteins found in animals with high biological value. The darker the buckwheat flour the more protein it contains.

BUCKWHEAT ALSO RICH IN MINERALS & VITAMINS

While buckwheat contains this high amount of good biological protein, it is also high in manganese. Manganese is an important mineral to life and health. When it is deficient in the diet, many species of animals show postural skeletal defects. Nutritional researches prove that these defects are related to the reduction in the content of chondroitin in the tissue. This is a substance that resembles cartilage. Vitally needed for maintaining sound body structure, manganese is also essential for muscle control, reproductive systems, health growth, good metabolism and the activation of enzymes.

There is no grain as rich in rutin as buckwheat. Rutin is one of the bioflavonoids that is so vital in helping to reduce capillary fragility. The rutin in buckwheat gives the best possible protection for maintaining sound blood vessels.

Magnesium, which is found abundantly in buckwheat, is an exceptionally rich mineral so essential to human health. Magnesium is vital as an activator of enzymes through which we use both vitamins and protein. It is known nutritionally as the spark plug which starts the chain reaction that metabolizes food.

HERE'S HOW TO SERVE BUCKWHEAT

Buckwheat may be prepared and served in many tasty and delicious ways. In rural Europe the peasants mix boiled buckwheat groats, or kasha, with a wide variety of other foods such as mushrooms, chopped onions and eggs. Buckwheat groats are delicious when eaten as a cereal and can also be used in puddings and cakes.

Buckwheat is a staple food used abundantly in the diet of the Japanese people. One of the most tasty and delicious ways they have of preparing buckwheat is in the form of noodles. The Japanese are absolutely famous for their buckwheat noodle soup. Many health food stores can supply you with buckwheat noodles.

As stated, buckwheat is sold in its natural state as groats. It can be purchased ground finely, medium or coarse. Following is a very simple recipe used in Europe:

EUROPEAN BUCKWHEAT (GROATS) RECIPE

In an iron pot or heavy stainless steel pan place one cup of groats. Add three cups of water, three tablespoons of oil, and two beaten whole eggs. Cover lid and let cook for 30 minutes over a medium flame, or until the mixture is thoroughly absorbed in the groats.

This is a standard recipe used in Romania, Bulgaria, Czechoslovakia, Russia, Yugoslavia and Poland.

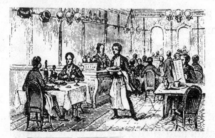

**BUCKWHEAT PANCAKES
ARE FAMOUS IN AMERICAN CUISINE**

Buckwheat pancakes and flapjacks have been a favorite of Americans for decades, especially in the winter. The buckwheat pancake has become so famous that we now have specialty restaurants known as pancake houses where many different recipes are used. Buckwheat pancakes can be served with a wide choice of delicious toppings . . . honey jelly or jam, honey fruit preserves, fresh bananas and other fruits, 100% maple syrup, melted salt free butter, honey, molasses, sour cream, and creamed cheese.

How well I remember when I was just a farm boy back in Virginia, pancakes tasted exquisite to me. One thing about farm life is that farmers earn their breakfast. At 4:30 in the morning we were up to feed the fowl, milk and feed the cattle, collect the eggs, chop the wood and perform the many other farm chores. At 7:00 o'clock sharp the breakfast bell rang and all hands rushed to the breakfast where steaming hot stacks of pungent buckwheat pancakes with all kinds of accessories such as honey, jam, jelly and molasses, awaited us.

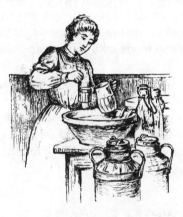

CAUTION
BUCKWHEAT
PANCAKES
CAN BE
FATTENING

As stated, buckwheat contains a tremendous amount of good biological protein, and the milk and eggs in the batter, fortify the protein. This in itself is good nutrition. But when the concentrated carbohydrates such as molasses, honey, syrup, jams, jellies and preserves are added, the carbohydrates count is considerably increased. Caution and discretion must be exercised in the amount of carbohydrates used or there will be a gain in body weight.

It is very important that the jams, jellies and preserves used on buckwheat cakes be made with honey rather than white sugar or raw sugar. Raw sugar, generally called turbinado sugar, is a washed sugar which has not been bleached nor refined and it is far preferable to the common white and bleached sugar. However, it is still a concentrated carbohydrate and can rapidly use up the body's insulin. Many natural diet conscious people consider raw sugar to be a natural product when in reality it is not, since much refinement goes on from the sugar cane to the production of raw sugar.

When too much raw sugar is used in the diet, it can produce a condition called "hypoglycemia" or low blood sugar. When there is insufficient insulin to handle concentrated sugars, a great inbalance takes place in the body. I must caution every health nutritional conscious person to use raw sugar with great discretion. There is not too great a difference between refined white sugar and raw sugar or brown sugar. Naturally, the insulin of the body can handle a small amount of raw sugar, but only a small amount. Personally, I do not have raw sugar in my kitchen and I do not prepare any foods with raw sugar. I always substitute honey.

Buckwheat pancakes may be eaten on special occasions, but they're not a food that should be a regular part of the menu. No matter how well you make a pancake, the digestive tract has to work very hard to digest it. That is the reason I feel there are better ways to use buckwheat such as in the form of buckwheat noodles and buckwheat groats.

BRAGG BUCKWHEAT PANCAKES

¾ c buckwheat flour	1¾ tsp double acting baking powder
¾ c raw wheat germ	2 eggs, lightly beaten
¼ c wholewheat flour	3 tbsp cold pressed oil such as soy, peanut, corn or safflour
3 tbsp honey or raw sugar	Water or milk, preferably certified raw milk.

In a bowl mix the buckwheat flour, raw wheat germ, whole wheat flour, honey or raw sugar and baking powder. Stir in the eggs, oil and enough milk or water to make a batter the consistency of thick, heavy cream. Ladle the mixture onto a hot, oiled griddle. When holes appear on the surface of the pancakes, turn to brown second side. Makes about 8 large pancakes.

If you have a favorite buckwheat pancake recipe containing no refined white sugar or refined white flour, or any other ingredient not inconsistent with good natural nutrition, you may use your own recipe. You can always substitute whole grain flour for refined flour. You can always substitute honey for refined white sugar.

USE NO SALT!—IT'S HARMFUL!

Most recipes for pancakes call for salt, either common table salt or sea salt. I do not use any kind of salt, whether it's regular salt or sea salt. They're both inorganic and can do irreparable damage to the body, in the retention of liquids as well as dehydration, and causing the natural moisture of the skin to evaporate.

The body is an organic instrument and can use or metabolize into blood, flesh, bones, fingernails and hair only that which is organic, that which is living or has lived.

So in your buckwheat pancake recipes and all recipes, eliminate the salt and sea salt, and that includes vegetized salt because vegetized salt is nothing more than common table salt with the addition of dehydrated vegetables. Salt is an enemy to the human body and should not be used.

You will continuously be told that in hot weather when the loss of sodium is high due to perspiration, that extra amounts of salt and salt tablets should be used. It isn't this inorganic sodium chloride the body needs, however. It is the organic sodium which is found abundantly in fruits and vegetables, celery being the highest carrier of high sodium content.

All soils are rich in inorganic sodium, so plants use the sodium they require and convert the inorganic sodium into organic sodium.

Be sure to include citrus fruits in your diet during hot weather, as these are also a prime source of Vitamin C. You need increased amounts of Vitamin C in order to help keep "cool"—it helps maintain body temperature at an even keel.

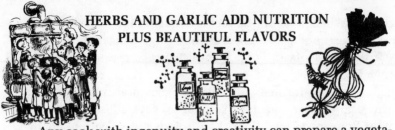

HERBS AND GARLIC ADD NUTRITION
PLUS BEAUTIFUL FLAVORS

Any cook with ingenuity and creativity can prepare a vegetable to be the rarest of foods in delicacy. There is no better way to discover the unsurpassed quality of fine foods than by experimenting with herb cookery in vegetables, by preparing them properly to conserve all the vitamins, minerals, and food values and by bringing out their true qualities of flavor pointed up by harmoniously blended seasoning. It is not necessary to have them rich and heavily spiced. They can be standard items of fine food, delicately flavored and served in entirely new ways designed to excite the palate with a new adventure.

Cooking with herbs is a delightful and healthful experience. Of all foods, herbs are designed to point up the flavor of vegetables more interestingly.

During my many years of food research, I have found garlic to be one of the greatest foods given to us by Mother Nature. In my opinion, it is the world's greatest natural antibiotic. It contains nutritional factors of great value that have never been isolated and discovered by nutritional science. Therefore, I have included garlic in many of my recipes for added zesty, delicious flavors.

The only indictment many people have against garlic is that it leaves an odor on the breath which they feel is offensive to others. I have been able to overcome the retaining of garlic on my breath by slowly chewing and insalivating a teaspoon of finely chopped parsley. The chlorophyl in any dark green vegetable will help absorb almost all odors from garlic or onions.

On the market today is a product called "Binaca" which can be purchased at drug stores. A drop of this on the tongue will cause the garlic or onion odor to immediately disappear. So there's no reason why you should not eat garlic and receive the tremendous nutritional benefits from this wonder herb.

40

DO NOT USE MONOSODIUM GLUTAMATE (MSG)

Read the label on foods carefully. Monosodium glutamate should not be used in your cooking at any time. It is the one flavor enhancer that has absolutely nothing good to offer in the way of nutrition. I believe in time when all the research is completed, that the Government will take it off the market.

Nutritional Scientists have learned in laboratory experiments that monosodium glutamate induces convulsive disorders in rats. Scientists injected MSG into the stomachs of adult rats and found that 31% of the animals experienced spastic tremors, 17% suffered seizures, and 29 of the 119 rats studied died within twenty-four hours after the injection.

The laboratory scientists further found that the feeding of MSG to rats caused a condition known as "spreading depression" by affecting the cerebral cortex of the brain, temporarily blocking some very important functions of that organ.

The scientists further found that migraine headaches in humans have been caused by eating food seasoned with MGS.

It is a fact that glutamate is naturally present in the brain, as well as in all body proteins, but too much of it in the nervous system can destroy nerve cells. (It is a known fact that nerve cells, once destroyed, can never be replaced.) Sodium is never normally present in the nervous system because of a barrier between the blood and the brain. This barrier is very selective and allows substances the brain needs, such as blood sugar, to pass through, and keeps others away.

Many people go throughout life committing partial suicide—destroying their health, youth, beauty, talents, energies, creative qualities. Indeed, to learn how to be good to oneself is often more difficult than to learn how to be good to others.

Whatsoever was the father of a disease; an ill diet was the mother.
— Herbert, 1859

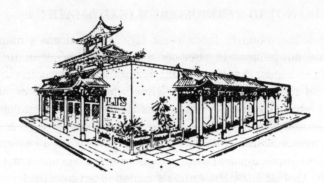

THE CHINESE RESTAURANT SYNDROME

Here in Honolulu, Hawaii, where I am writing this book, we have a large population of Oriental people and many of these Orientals are restaurant keepers. I live in one of the largest apartment and hotel buildings in Honolulu and have a chance to observe the effects of monosodium glutamate in people who eat Chinese food. Chinese restaurants use large amounts of monosodium glutamate and soy sauce, both of which are highly saturated with concentrated sodium.

Many doctors with whom I am acquainted with tell me that tourists and natives suffer adverse reactions while dining at Chinese restaurants. The reaction involves numbness in the back of the neck, general weakness, palpitation and headaches. MGS produces a flushing that is very uncomfortable while in progress in the body. I have personally seen people eating a Chinese meal, and within twenty minutes after the ingestion of the Chinese dishes suddenly develop a tightening of the face, associated with numbness. At times the mouth becomes so weak that chewing is impaired. A sensation of dizziness follows, associated with flushing and sweating. Many people complain of a band-like headache with orbital pain.

I personally saw a man digest a Chinese egg roll and within an hour have an attack of acute myocardial infarction; in other words, a heart attack. I have seen extreme fatigue develop in people who eat Chinese food, and also attacks of vomiting caused from the MSG in the Chinese dishes.

NO NUTRITIONAL VALUE IN MSG

On close examination we find MSG has absolutely no nutritional value. Then why do food manufacturers continually add MGS to foods? In my opinion, the answer is to make the product seem better than it is, masking its true lack of flavor. So the only actual value I see is the large revenues it brings to chemical companies.

It you're really interested in eating foods and enjoying their natural flavors, why settle for an artificial flavor that could cause irreparable damage to your nervous system?

Many times MGS is placed in common foods such as mayonnaise, French dressing and other salad dressings, enjoying the privileged status of a "permissable ingredient" not required to be declared on the label. That is the reason I believe all kinds of prepared and processed foods should be avoided on a natural diet unless they come from the health food stores. Even then, labels should be read and questions asked as to whether the foods they are selling contain MGS.

In my opinion, the MGS contained in baby food is a crime against a child too young to defend itself against the ravages of monosodium glutamate. MGS comes under many trade names and that is the reason I say again "read the labels." If the products contain MGS, don't eat them.

You do not need flavor enhancers when you eat natural food. There's plenty of true food taste in natural health foods which cannot be improved by the adding of MGS or any other flavor enhancer.

Many prepared, canned and packaged vegetarian products have had MGS added and I've seen vegetarians, who are conscientiously trying to lead a good nutritional health life, become desperately ill from these foods. So if the products contain MGS, drop them—they're not for you—they have no health value whatsoever.

"To preserve health is a moral and religious duty, for health is the basis for all social virtues. We can no longer be useful when not well."
— **Dr. Samuel Johnson, Father of Dictionaries**

BRAGG LIQUID AMINOS

ADDS DELICIOUS FLAVOR TO MANY OF THESE RECIPES
For Extra Hi-Protein Flavoring and Zest To Your Meals
Bragg Liquid Aminos is Delicious
to Enhance The Natural Flavors.

All vegetable source - with natural flavoring, contains no preservatives. It has a meat-like, savory flavor, yet contains no meat or meat products.

WHAT ARE AMINO ACIDS? They are the link between the protein you eat and your body tissue. They are carried by your bloodstream to every part of your body where they set to work repairing, building and maintaining the all important body tissues.

Be sure your high protein food
is a quality one by checking these points:
- It must be completely natural.
- It must give you its strength or potency by listing the number of Amino Acids on the label.
- It must taste delicious for added zest to the diet.
- It must be made under the strictest standards to preserve its natural amino acids.

Bragg Liquid Aminos meets all these high standards and is an outstanding addition to many of these meatless recipes for it gives you extra nutrients and delicious flavoring.

BRAGG LIQUID AMINOS
has a way of making these foods taste just a little better...

- vegetables ● brown rice ● beans of all kinds ● vegetable burgers
- soups ● casseroles ● gravies and sauces ● salad dressings

Bragg Liquid Aminos contain the following Amino Acids,
the building blocks of the body.

*Lysine	Serine	*Valine
Histidine	Glutamic Acid	*Methionine
Arginine	Proline	*Isoleucine
*Tryptophan	Glycine	*Leucine
Aspartic Acid	Alanine	Tyrosine
*Threonine	Cystine	*Phenylalanine

*essential Amino Acids in naturally associated amounts as derived from a specially formulated liquid-form of vegetable protein.

(continued on page 66)

MUSHROOMS
AN ANCIENT NUTRITIONAL
DELICACY

Egyptian hieroglyphics over 5,000 years ago recorded legends showing belief that the mushroom was the plant of immortality. Japanese legend has it that one variety of mushroom can prolong life. The ancient Chinese believed that it was an aphrodisiac. The Pharaohs of Egypt were so fascinated with the delicious flavor of mushroom, that they decreed that no commoner could ever touch a mushroom, thus assuring themselves of the entire supply.

The epicures of Rome, the royalty of Britain and France all permitted only the courts and the palaces to serve mushrooms.

Advanced civilizations in many parts of the world—Mexico, Central America, Russia, Greece, China and Egypt, practiced mushroom rituals. Many believed that mushrooms contained properties which would confer the ability to find lost objects, heal the sick, produce supernatural strength and aid the soul in reaching the realm of the gods.

MUSHROOMS—A NATURAL "WONDER FOOD"

The mushroom actually is one of nature's wonder foods. It isn't a vegetable, a nut, a seed, an animal, a fruit or grain. It manufactures no green chlorophyl, needs no sunlight, yet grows with great rapidity. Some varieties are even reputed to have anti-cholesterol and antibiotic properties. The most common variety is brimful of protein of a high quality as well as the B-vitamins.

Many people think of mushrooms as garnishes, but these tasty morsels, in fact, make a wonderful health food. They contain a great deal of pantothenic acid (B-5), many times called

45

the anti-stress vitamin because it keeps the bodily processes running smoothly in the face of terrific shocks to the system. It is also important to the production of anti-bodies to protect against infection and has been used with great success to minimize allergic reactions.

The mushroom is a greater storehouse of Vitamin B-5 (pantothenic acid) than any other plant food that grows. Mushrooms are also a great source of niacin (B-3) which, among numerous other protective roles, keeps cholesterol levels in check and promotes the wellbeing of the central nervous system, including mental health.

Generous amounts of riboflavin (B-2) are found in the mushroom. Riboflavin is needed to spark many vital enzyme reactions, to help keep the skin youthful looking and healthy, and to help repair injuries. The mushroom contains useful amounts of thiamine (B-1) and pyridoxine (B-6). The mushroom can be called a splendid blood builder as it contains a goodly amount of iron and copper.

On one of my hiking trips in Canada, I became stranded in the north woods where I lived seventeen days in good health on the wild mushrooms. I never lost my energy because the mushroom contains many vitamins and minerals as well as splendid protein, fats and carbohydrates.

The mushroom has other nutritional pluses, one being the high content in glutamic acid, the amino acid so necessary to the proper functioning of the brain.

The mushroom is delicious, both raw and cooked. The fresh mushrooms are preferable to the canned because the canned mushrooms contain only half the amount of the nutrients of the fresh, and approximately 70% less thiamine. Salt is added to canned mushrooms and much of the delicate flavor is lost. In my opinion, the best, the simplest and the most nutritious way to eat mushrooms is raw. For those who have never had the delight of eating raw mushrooms, the flavor may come as a delicious surprise.

Accuse not nature, she hath done her part; do thou but thine.
—Milton, Paradise Lost

The mushroom may be used in salads and may be added to any casseroles, vegetarian dishes, soups, and health sandwiches. Here is my favorite sandwich recipe:

MUSHROOM DELIGHT SANDWICH

On one slice of 100% whole grain bread, toasted, place the following: Health mayonnaise, sliced fresh mushrooms, alfalfa sprouts, sunflower seeds, natural cheddar cheese, Swiss or Jack cheese, and sliced tomatoes. Instead of another piece of whole grain toast, top the sandwich with green lettuce leaves.

Many times I make variations of this sandwich. For example, I'll use onions or chopped green peppers, cucumbers or radishes. All you need is a little imagination and you can prepare many varieties of sandwiches which are meals within themselves because they have the nutrients for health building, and especially protein.

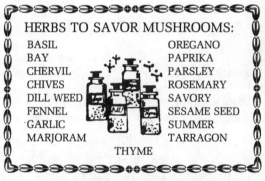

HERBS TO SAVOR MUSHROOMS:

BASIL	OREGANO
BAY	PAPRIKA
CHERVIL	PARSLEY
CHIVES	ROSEMARY
DILL WEED	SAVORY
FENNEL	SESAME SEED
GARLIC	SUMMER
MARJORAM	TARRAGON

THYME

MUSHROOM HERB SAUCE

1 c Mushrooms, fresh	2 tbsp butter salt-free
½ tsp Italian herbs	1 tbsp soya flour
1½ c Soya or Cow's Milk	1 tsp Bragg Liquid Aminos

Wash and chop mushrooms and stalks finely. Heat butter in pan, add flour and soya and stir well over gentle heat. Gradually add milk in small quantities, stirring briskly, till a smooth sauce results. Add mushrooms and simmer for 10 minutes.

I have told you the nutritional benefits of the buckwheat and that it is rich in protein and rutin. Here is one of my favorite buckwheat mushroom recipes:

BUCKWHEAT GROATS OR KASHA WITH MUSHROOMS

1 c buckwheat groats (often referred to as kasha)	2 tbsp oil (cold-pressed)
	2 c water
	1 or more cloves garlic (use garlic press)
2 raw eggs, beaten	
1 c mushrooms, sliced	1 tsp Bragg Aminos

Beat the eggs well and add the groats. Mix thoroughly to coat the grains. Brown mixture gently in oil (use a heavy skillet). Add the sliced mushrooms. Bring water to a boil and add the mixture together with the Bragg Aminos. Mix well and cook very slowly, covered, until all the liquid is absorbed and the kasha is light and fluffy.

MUSHROOM RICE

2 c brown rice, cooked	1½ c mushrooms, fresh
4 oz Cheddar cheese, grated	2 onions, chopped
½ tsp Italian Seasoning	2 eggs
	Soy Oil
1 tbsp Bragg Liquid Aminos	1 tsp Brewer's yeast

Wash and cook the rice in boiling water till tender. Peel and chop the onions and saute in soy oil till golden. Wash and roughly chop the mushrooms and add to the onions in the last five minutes of cooking. Beat the eggs and mix with the grated cheese, seasoning and Brewer's yeast, onions and mushrooms and rice. Place in a greased baking dish. Bake in 400° oven for 30-40 minutes.

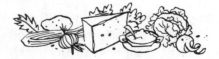

STUFFED MUSHROOMS—BROILED

⅓ c cold-pressed oil
½ c raw wheat germ
2 tbsp minced parsley
2 tbsp minced onions
  Garlic optional
14 large mushrooms (remove stems and set aside)

3 tbsp chopped sunflower seeds
1 tbsp Bragg Aminos
2 tbsp grated cheddar cheese

Finely chop the mushroom stems. Add the remaining ingredients and mix well. Top the mushroom caps with this mixture and sprinkle with chopped or whole sunflower seeds. Lightly broil in pie tin until the caps are tender.

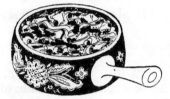

MUSHROOM BARLEY GOULASH

2 c sliced mushrooms
2 c diced carrots
2 c diced celery
½ c diced green pepper
1 c diced onion
1 c natural whole unpearled barley

⅓ c cold-pressed oil
1 c diced tomatoes
2 tbsp Bragg Aminos
3 cloves chopped garlic

Cover barley with water, add garlic, herbs and Aminos. Cover and cook on low flame for 1-1½ hours until almost done, stirring occasionally. Heat the oil in a large kettle and lightly saute the carrots, celery, green pepper, garlic and onion for 3 minutes. Now add the cooked barley and the remainder of ingredients and finish cooking—takes about 10-15 minutes if you enjoy vegetables not overdone.

Variations: You can vary this recipe by adding various vegetables as you have them on hand or add more water and this turns into a delicious, thick soup. You may enjoy it as a casserole with grated cheese sprinkled over the top just before serving.

SAUTEED MUSHROOMS ON WHOLE GRAIN TOAST

Wash mushrooms thoroughly. Separate the large from the small ones, cutting the large mushrooms down the center of the stem. Saute in a heavy skillet, using 2 tbsp. unsalted butter and a generous amount of cold-pressed oil (I prefer olive oil), the following: Mushrooms, chopped garlic (optional), 1 tsp. Bragg Aminos and ½ tsp. lemon juice. Gently stir with wooden spoon and when done, arrange generous amounts on toasted whole grain bread, adding some of the sauce from the sauteed mixture.

MUSHROOM BURGERS

2 c finely chopped mushrooms	1 small onion, finely chopped
1 egg	1 tsp Bragg Aminos

1 c toasted whole wheat bread crumbs (dextronized or melba toast which has been placed in 275° oven until thoroughly dried)

Mix well and form into small burgers. Saute in oil, turning to brown on both sides.

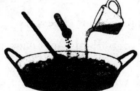

MUSHROOM-CHEESE OMELET

1 c mushrooms cut in half, stemwise	⅓ c cheddar cheese, finely grated
4 eggs	4 tbsp top milk or cream
1 clove garlic, optional	1 tsp Bragg Aminos

Saute mushrooms in oil and a tsp. of butter, add Bragg Aminos, garlic, eggs, milk and grated cheese. Be sure to keep the heat low as you want the omelet to be a golden brown, but not burned. When omelet solidifies on top, gently turn with spatula and brown other side.

PROTEIN MUSHROOM LOAF

2 c finely chopped
mushrooms
1/3 c chopped onions
1/3 c chopped green
peppers
1/2 c tomatoes
2 c toasted whole wheat
bread crumbs

1/2 c grated natural cheddar
cheese
1 tbsp Bragg Aminos
1/3 c sunflower seeds,
chopped
1/3 c walnuts, chopped
2 eggs
2 cloves garlic, optional

Mix all the ingredients together and bake in greased loaf pan
30 minutes in moderate oven (375°).

BROWN RICE MUSHROOM LOAF

2 c cooked brown rice
1 c chopped mushrooms
2 eggs
1/2 c grated natural cheddar cheese

1/2 c minced onions
1/3 c sunflower seeds,
chopped

Combine all the ingredients and pack in greased casserole.
Bake 30 minutes in moderate oven (375°).

SERBIAN MUSHROOM VEGETABLE GOULASH

1 c chopped mushrooms
1 c chopped onions
1 c chopped sweet green
peppers
1 c coarsely sliced green or red cabbage
2 tbsp cold-pressed oil (This recipe I prefer olive oil)

1 tbsp Bragg Aminos
1 c chopped tomatoes
2 cloves garlic (optional)
1 c grated beets

Mix all the ingredients together. Place in greased baking pan
and bake 30 minutes in moderate oven or until done.

HI-PROTEIN MUSHROOM STUFFING
FOR BAKED POTATO
Makes 4 stuffed halves

½ c finely chopped
   sauteed mushrooms
⅓ c natural cheddar
½ c finely chopped green onions with stems

1 tbsp oil or unsalted
   butter per potato
⅓ tsp kelp seasoning

Bake large Russet potato or potatoes. (Scrub thoroughly so that skins can be eaten as many important nutrients, and particularly protein, are contained in the skins of potatoes.)

When baked, cut in half and with a spoon scoop out the inside, leaving ¼ of the potato against the skin. In a mixing bowl mash thoroughly the potato, or potatoes, and add the remainder of the ingredients, allowing 1 tbsp. of cold-pressed oil or 1 tbsp. unsalted butter for each potato. Replace this mixture in the potato shells, sprinkle with paprika and bake 10 minutes or until cheese has melted.

MUSHROOM ZUCCHINI-CHEESE CASSEROLE

3 c zucchini cut into ½"
   slices
1 c chopped fresh
   mushrooms
2 eggs, lightly beaten
1 onion, finely chopped
⅓ c cold-pressed oil
1 c natural brown rice, cooked

1 tbsp Bragg Aminos
2 large cloves garlic,
   pressed (optional)
⅓ tsp marjoram
⅓ c grated Parmesan
   cheese
¾ c raw wheat germ
1 c cottage cheese

Mix thoroughly all ingredients in large mixing bowl. Put in greased casserole, bake 45 minutes or until done in a 375° oven.

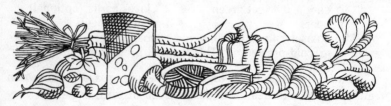

VEGETARIAN MUSHROOM CUTLETS

1 c chopped fresh
  mushrooms
½ c finely grated raw beets
½ c grated fresh carrots
¾ c chopped onions
2 tbsp Bragg Aminos

2 eggs, well beaten
½ c sunflower seeds,
  finely ground
⅓ tsp caraway seeds
½ c raw wheat germ

Combine entire mixture in mixing bowl and mix well. If mixture is too wet to form into patties, add more wheat germ. Place mixture in refrigerator for 30 minutes. Shape into patties. Saute in lightly oiled skillet until brown; turn to brown the other side.

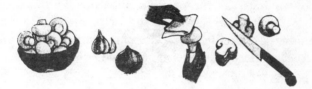

MUSHROOM LENTIL BURGERS

1 c finely chopped
  mushrooms
2 c cooked lentils
1 c toasted whole wheat
  bread crumbs
½ c raw wheat germ
½ c finely chopped parsley

¾ c finely chopped onions
½ tsp celery seed
3 tbsp oil
1 tbsp Bragg Aminos
1 clove garlic, pressed
  (optional)

Mash lentils lightly. Add remainder of ingredients. Form the mixture into patties. Coat or roll in finely ground whole wheat crumbs or flour. Heat the oil in a skillet and saute the patties on both sides until brown.

The Doctor of the future will give no medicine but will interest his patients in the care of the human frame in diet and in the cause and prevention of disease.

—Thomas A. Edison

MUSHROOM SOYBEAN PATTIES

1 c chopped mushrooms	½ c raw wheat germ
1½ c cooked soybeans	¼ c cottage cheese
2 eggs, lightly beaten	1 tbsp Bragg Aminos
½ c finely chopped onions	⅛ tsp dry mustard
½ c non-fat dry milk solids	½ c sesame seeds

Mash soybeans to a fine pulp in a mixing bowl. Add all other ingredients and mix well. If mixture is too dry, add small amounts of hot water until it can be shaped into patties. Before sauteeing, dry for 15 minutes; then saute patties until both sides are brown.

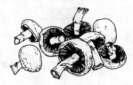

STUFFED MUSHROOMS

12 large or 35 small mushrooms	¼ c wheat germ or whole wheat bread crumbs
3 tbsp soy oil	
1 tsp shallot or garlic, minced	1 tsp Bragg Aminos
	2 tbsp vegetable broth
2 tsp onion, minced	2 tbsp Romano or Parmesan Cheese, grated
1 tbsp parsley, minced	

Snap off mushroom stems and mince fine. Heat butter and 1 tablespoon of the oil in a skillet. Add minced mushroom, shallot and parsley. Cook until lightly browned. Stir in wheat germ or crumbs, Bragg Aminos and enough broth to make a mixture which clings together. Arrange mushroom caps, cup side up, in a greased shallow baking dish. Fill with crumb mixture. Brush with oil and sprinkle with cheese. Bake at 400°, 10 to 15 mins.

Health is the soul which animates all enjoyment of life.

—Temple

SESAME SEEDS
A POWERHOUSE OF NUTRITION

As I have told you, I have been a world traveler for over 60 years. And I have been to the faraway places—Asia Minor, the back country of Brazil, Turkey and Greece. In practically every country, the sesame seed has been a standard item of food. In these countries I have watched this hairy-leaf plant, with its crimped edge buds, turning to pale pink blossoms and as fall approached, the four-sided velvety sesame seed pods developing almost ready for the magic "popping day". Suddenly one by one the light green oblong pods of the sesame started to pop. I would take a paper bag and catch the honey-colored seeds as they broke forth from their sheaths. I felt like saying, "Open, Sesame" because sesame seeds have magic.

Four hundred years before the birth of Christ, the great physician Hippocrates used the sesame seed in his healing compounds. Greek soldiers carried a bag of sesame seeds for their emergency rations — they realized the high food value of this magic food.

SESAME SEEDS WERE LOVED BY THE ANCIENTS

So ancient is the sesame plant that history tells us the ancient gods of the Assyrians drank sesame wine to give them strength and endurance when they began creating the world.

I have visited Egyptian tombs, dating back more than 4,000 years, depicting a baker adding sesame seeds to his dough.

Chinese documents mention the seed in the fifth century. Right here in the United States, early in the 19th century, the great patriot Thomas Jefferson became excited over the potential value of the sesame seed. He thought it would help the farmers if they cultivated this magic plant.

It is true that the sesame plant is cultivated all over the world and is a very important item of food, but in Java it grows wild, and botanists agree that the plant must have originated in the Sunda Islands off the coast of Java and Sumatra.

All over the world you will find different races eating the sesame seed and using sesame oil for cooking because it does not readily become rancid.

Today most of the sesame seeds are imported to the United States from the South American countries.

SESAME SEEDS AND SESAME OIL— POPULAR IN THE UNITED STATES

Last year the United States imported 45,000,000 pounds of sesame seeds and 2,108,000 pounds of sesame oil, most of it coming from the South American countries. Nutritionally, the sesame seed ranks high. First, it is high in protein the body can use. It is high in magnesium (a nutrient deficient in most diets in the USA) which has been proved to combat chronic fatigue.

The sesame seed contains a high amount of lecithin which helps combat the deadly waxy cholesterol which forms in the arteries. It has an abundance of calcium, vitamins C, E and F.

Sesame Seeds Are Not Only A Nutritional Addition To Foods But The Almond Flavor Is Delicate And Delicious.

THE SECRET OF USING SESAME SEEDS

Let me give you a word of warning. If you are going to use the sesame seeds in the recipe mixture, toast them first.

The method of toasting is as follows: Scatter the seeds on a baking tray and toast for 10 to 15 minutes in a 300° oven, or until the seeds are a light golden brown.

If you are going to use the seeds as toppers where the food will be baked or broiled, there's no need to toast them first. Because of their delightful, delicate almond-like flavor, sesame seeds can be used as a piquant addition to almost any food—raw salads, soups, entrees, vegetarian loaves and vegetarian patties, to even health candy.

Personally, I like to sprinkle toasted sesame seeds on my vegetable salads. At the end of my meal, I enjoy the delicious flavor of sesame seed cookies. To any of your favorite cookie recipes simply add sesame seeds and you'll find they're delicious. The following recipe is a favorite of mine:

PEANUT BUTTER SESAME BALLS

½ c honey
¾ c powdered skim milk
2 tbsp boiling water
¾ c natural raw, unsalted non-hydrogenated peanut butter
(buy in health store)

1 c uncooked rolled oats
¾ c toasted sesame seeds
1 tsp pure vanilla extract

Combine all ingredients and form into balls. Roll balls with generous amounts of sesame seeds. These are delicious without baking or you can bake in low oven for 10 minutes.

SESAME SEEDS GO WITH EVERYTHING

When making sandwiches sprinkle on a generous amount of toasted sesame seeds. I can think of hardly any food with which sesame seeds cannot be used. I find that the delicate almond-like flavor of toasted sesame seeds is delicious on health iced desserts such as cakes and pies.

TAHINI—FAMOUS ARABIAN RECIPE RICH IN PROTEIN

Tahini is actually sesame seed butter, the seed having been crushed into a delectable paste. It has all the nutritional values of the whole seed and is versatile in its use in cooking, baking, in sandwiches and desserts.

The Arabs originated Tahini hundreds of years ago and here is a famous recipe used all over the Arab world:

TAHINI PROTEIN SPREAD

2 c cooked garbanzos 1 lemon
1 tsp Bragg Aminos   2 cloves garlic (optional)
1 c Tahini (purchased at your health food store)

In blender place the cooked garbanzos with enough liquid to keep it dry about the consistency of peanut butter. Add 1 c Tahini, juice of 1 lemon and 1 tsp. Bragg Aminos. Blend well and chill one hour before serving. This makes a delicious and nutritious sandwich spread, as well as a delightful and tasty dip to which I often add several cloves of pressed garlic. This combination is very important on a vegetarian diet since it supplies such a tremendous amount of protein.

HULLED MILLET
IT'S FOOD AND PROTEIN VALUE

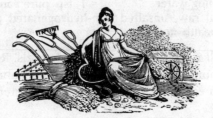

Millet has formed an important part of the food of man for eons of time. It carries a high percentage of protein, as well as calcium, phosphorous, lecithin, iron, potassium, thiamine, riboflaven and niacin. Millet is an exceptionally easily digested alkaline grain. It can be used as a cereal or in soups or casseroles. Here are two favorite recipes of mine:

HOT MILLET CEREAL

½ c millet
1 c water
yogurt

Dates, raisins, or
figs
honey

Bring 2 c. water to boil in heavy pan with a tight lid. Stir in ½ c millet and continue stirring to boil Cover and cook over low heat 35 - 40 minutes. Dates, raisins, or figs may be added the last 5 minutes of cooking time. Serve with yogurt and honey. This makes a complete meal in itself.

MILLET CASSEROLE

2 c water
1 c hulled millet
½ c chopped celery
½ tbsp Bragg Aminos
2 cloves pressed garlic
(optional)

⅓ tsp poultry seasoning
½ c chopped onion
1 c chopped mushrooms
½ c sunflower seeds
1 c chopped zuccchini or
yellow squash

Mix ingredients well. Pour into a casserole and bake at 300° for 1-1½ hours until done.

58

BARLEY
A GOOD SOURCE OF PROTEIN

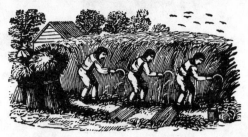

Barley is a very ancient food. In Biblical times all bread was made from whole natural unpearled barley. The Phoenicians, the Egyptians, the early Greeks, the Romans and the Israelites used barley extensively in their diets.

Barley can be used in soups, vegetarian meatloafs, and soaked for an hour and cooked as a main dish, seasoned with unsalted butter or oil.

Here is our favorite vegetable barley soup recipe:

BRAGG VEGETABLE BARLEY SOUP

1 c chopped onions	2 c diced yellow squash
1 c chopped celery	2 c cauliflower florets
1 c minced fresh parsley	2 tomatoes
1 c sliced mushrooms	1 tbsp Bragg Aminos
1 c diced carrots	2 qts water
½ c unpearled barley that's been soaked one hour	½ tsp Italian Herb Seasonings

In a large soup kettle saute onions, celery and garlic in oil for 3 minutes. Add mushrooms and continue to saute. Add water, barley and other ingredients. Cook for 45 minutes or until done. Serve in soup bowls and garnish with sunflower and sesame seed meal. This garnish adds deliciousness and also fortifies the soup with protein.

"Living under conditions of modern life, it is important to bear in mind that the preparation and refinement of food products either entirely eliminates or in part destroys the vital elements in the original material."

— U.S. Dept. of Agriculture

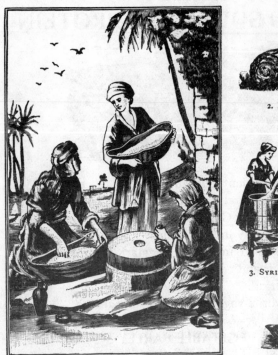

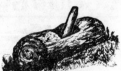

2. INDIAN MILL.

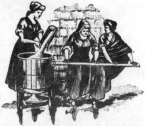

3. SYRIAN MILL.

1. ORIENTAL MILL.

4. MEXICAN MILL.

ANCIENT METHODS OF GRINDING GRAINS AND SEEDS

These methods retained the whole goodness for perfect health and vitality. Today modern milling removes most or all of the vital nutrients to maintain long shelf life of the products. Now the alert health minded people are grinding their own grains and seeds as they are needed, thereby getting all the precious vitamins, minerals and nutrients so important to health and long-life. Vitamin "E" that is so essential to health is present in freshly ground grains and seeds. Hand and electric grinders and mills are available at most Health Stores.

60

CHINESE YOGURT OR TOFU A POWERHOUSE OF NUTRITIONAL PROTEIN

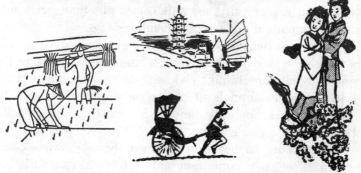

Many years ago when I was an associate editor of Bernarr Macfadden's famous Physical Culture Magazine, I made one of the greatest nutritional discoveries of my life.

Mr. Macfadden and I had heard of the tremendous vitality, energy and health of the people of Manchuria, China and it was decided I should do the research on these amazing people. In those days of no airplanes, the trip to Manchuria was a long and arduous one. But I was well rewarded because it was there that I discovered the magic of the soybean, the most potent of vegetable high-protein foods.

The people of Manchuria were beautiful—the women exquisite. Never have I seen the figures and faces with such wonderful skin and muscle tone—no over-weights and no under-weights. What intrigued me the most was their healthy and beautiful children. After being weaned, the children are put on soy milk because Manchuria is not a dairy country; in fact, they had very few cows. Cows, being good mainly for producing milk, were too specialized for the Manchurians. They were also too expensive because a cow eats five times the calories that it delivers as milk, and ten times the calories it returns as meat. Animals of any kind were not numerous in Manchuria, when you considered the large area of the country and the great number of people.

As stated, instead of cow's milk, the Manchurians use soy milk. An acre of land can produce much more soy milk than it can produce cow's milk. Soy milk also has the advantage of being lower on the food chain, which means there is less contamination. Ecologically, soy milk is far better than cow's milk and has important nutritional advantages also.

The Manchurians make soy milk by grinding soybeans that have been soaked in water for 24 hours, then straining the remaining mixture through cheesecloth. The rough part of the beans is fed to animals or otherwise disposed of, and the "milk" remains. Soy milk, though, is almost never used as is, the way we use cow's milk.

For one thing, soybeans should never be eaten raw because uncooked soybeans contain an anti-nutritional factor that inhibits digestion of the enzyme trypsin.

The practice of the Manchurians is to precipitate the solids in soy milk by cooking it and then mixing in gypsum, which is calcium sulfate. The solids drop to the bottom of the container and the liquid is filtered off the top. When the moisture is pressed from the solids, the resulting food is called bean curd, bean cake, dom foo yuen (Chinese) or tofu (Japanese).

There is a close parallel between the process of making tofu and that of making yogurt. While soy milk is precipitated with magnesium sulfate, or sometimes calcium sulfate, yogurt is fermented by bacteria, especially Lacto Bacillus Bulgaricus.

When I first started eating tofu in Manchuria, it resembled yogurt so much that I called it "Chinese yogurt" in my writings.

Tofu can supply all the proteins the body needs in a vegetable form and it can be thoroughly enjoyed. Here in Hawaii where I live, delicious protein-packed tofu can be purchased in any super-market or health food store.

Tofu has a very close relationship to spun soy protein, currently the important food to replace meat. Many of you probably have already eaten spun protein mixed in with sausages or hamburger without knowing it. Today many institutional cafeterias and restaurants use spun protein mixed with meat as a meat extender.

I believe as the price of meat rises, tofu will be easy to obtain at the health food stores and supermarkets all over the United States. You can purchase canned tofu in the health food stores where it is called "soybean cheese". If you live in the city where there is a Chinese grocery, you can obtain fresh tofu daily.

Our favorite ways of eating tofu are: with chop suey, in vegetable casseroles and scrambled with eggs. Here is the Bragg favorite chop suey recipe:

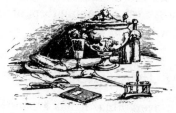

CHOP SUEY WITH TOFU

1 c celery (sliced on the bias or slantwise)	1 small can water chest-nuts, sliced†
1 c chopped onions	1 small can bamboo shoots†
1 c chopped green pepper	¼ c cold-pressed oil
1 c finely shredded or grated carrots	2 tbsp Bragg Aminos
½ tsp Chinese Five Spice* (Schilling or Spice Island)	2 cloves chopped garlic (optional)
1 c Mung bean sprouts†	1 c canned or fresh mushrooms
1 c Tofu	

*Note: This is found on the herb or seasoning shelf of your food market.

†Note: If these cannot be purchased fresh, they can always be found in cans in supermarkets.

The Chinese never over-cook their vegetables. They use a round pan for sauteeing their vegetables called the "wok" or a heavy iron skillet.

Place oil, Bragg Aminos and Chinese Five Spice in skillet under low heat until the oil is hot, but not bubbling. Then add all the ingredients, except the tofu and the mung bean sprouts (these are not put in until the last thing). Use a wooden spoon to continusously saute the vegetables (over not too intense heat), this kind of sauteeing retains all of the valuable vitamins, minerals, enzymes and nutrients. After the mixture is thoroughly heated (about ten minutes), gently place the tofu in the skillet and mix with the vegetables, being careful not to break up the little squares of tofu.

After the tofu has been thoroughly warmed with the vegetables, add a cup of fresh or canned mung bean sprouts. Serve with natural brown rice. To enhance the protein content of this meal, add to each serving a heaping tbsp. of almonds (slightly roast in oven, then sliver or slice).

VEGETABLE CASSEROLES USING TOFU

Tofu goes with everything. It has a neutral flavor, is very porous and absorbs the flavor of any food with which it is combined. Therefore, it can be mixed in with any casserole. For instance, if you are steaming broccoli, when almost done add 1 c. tofu cut into ½" squares.

Tofu can be cooked with string beans, tomatoes, peas, carrots, celery; in fact, any vegetable. The tofu will fortify the cooked vegetable. Remember, soybeans pack into their little round shells the most and the highest quality protein of just about any vegetable food. Nutrition-wise, soy beans are the greatest.

Learn the art of blending tofu with cooked vegetables, brown rice, seeds and nuts to make non-meat foods nutritionally and taste-wise as good as meat. Beans, natural brown rice, and tofu are a great protein combination. As a good guide to food combinations for high quality protein, blend in one meal as many vegetarian proteins as you can. For instance, to your casseroles, cooked vegetables and scrambled eggs you could add sunflower seeds.

The first wealth is health. Sickness is poor spirited and cannot serve anyone.
—Emerson

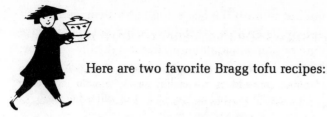

Here are two favorite Bragg tofu recipes:

TOFU CASSEROLE SUPREME

1-2 c tofu cut in 1" squares
 1 c peeled fresh tomatoes
 1 c chopped green pepper
 1 c sliced celery
 ¼ c cold-pressed oil or
 1 tbsp unsalted butter
 1 tsp Bragg Instant
        Vegetable Broth Powder

 1 c zucchini or crook neck
      squash
 1 c chopped onion
 1 tbsp Bragg Aminos
 ½ c chopped parsley
 2 cloves chopped garlic
      (optional)

Combine ingredients. Place casserole and bake 45 minutes or until almost done, in 375° oven. Then add 1 or 2 c. tofu and gently stir with wooden spoon, not breaking tofu squares, and bake 10 minutes longer. Serve with grated parmesan cheese.

TOFU AND SCRAMBLED EGGS

 3 eggs
 ½ c sliced onions (dry or
      green)
 2 cloves garlic (optional)

 ½ c chopped parsley
 1-2 c tofu cut in ½" squares
 1 tbsp Bragg Aminos
 ⅓ c parmesan cheese

In heavy skillet place 3 tbsp. cold-pressed oil or 1 tbsp. unsalted butter. Saute garlic and onions until onions become transparent. Add 3 well beaten eggs into which you have gently stirred the tofu, parsley and Bragg Aminos. Gently cook on one side, then turn with spatula to cook on the other until both sides are a golden brown. Sprinkle on parmesan cheese when served.

Now I see the secret of the making of the best persons, it is to grow in the open air, and eat and sleep with the earth.

— Walt Whitman

SUGGESTIONS FOR USING BRAGG LIQUID AMINOS

(continued from page 44)

AMINOS BROTH - one to two tablespoons Bragg Liquid Aminos to one cup hot water, or add to vegetable juices (tomato, celery or other juices). Flavor with minced onion, chives or other herbs.

AMINOS GRAVY - 1 tbsp Aminos, ¼ tsp Bragg Kelp Seasoning, 4 tbsp whole wheat flour, 4 tbsp melted salt-free butter, 2 cups water. Brown whole wheat flour in melted butter; add Aminos and Kelp; gradually stir in water and simmer until thickened.

IMPROVE SAUCES, SOUPS, CASSEROLES, VEGETABLES - Stir in Aminos ¼ tsp at a time until desired flavor is obtained.

USE ON SALADS AND OTHER FOODS - Blend a few dashes of Aminos into your favorite salad dressing. Sprinkle lightly on foods to enhance the natural taste.

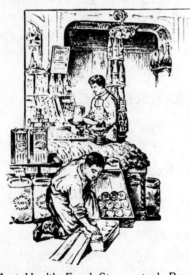

PURCHASE

BRAGG LIQUID AMINOS

AT YOUR LOCAL

HEALTH FOOD STORE

Most Health Food Stores stock Bragg Liquid Aminos...if they do not stock this wonderful product ask the store manager to order it from their distributor for you. If there are no Health Stores in your area and it's impossible to obtain - you may send direct to:

Live Food Products, Inc. **Desert Hot Springs, California 92240 U.S.A.**

For 16 ounces of Bragg Liquid Aminos send $1.99, plus $1.00 to cover postage, handling and insurance.

MEXICO
GIVES US DELICIOUS
MEATLESS PROTEIN DISHES

Most of the Mexican vegetarian dishes are composed of natural ground cornmeal, both white and yellow. Along with the corn is used cheese, fresh vegetables, chili powder, and pinto beans.

I have made several nutritional research expeditions into various parts of Mexico and have found that when the Mexican people lived on their simple, primitive, wholesome diet they enjoyed perfect health and had an abundance of energy. Their energy is shown in their vigorous dances, their splendid horsemanship and their tremendous endurance in carrying heavy loads on their backs for long distances at a time.

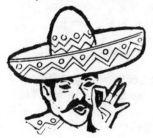

NOURISHING

MEXICAN RECIPES

Here's our Bragg favorite Mexican recipes:

TOSTADA

Place tortilla in a heavy skillet that has been lightly brushed with oil. Turn with spatula until thoroughly warm. Remove and place on plate. Heap refried pinto beans (see above recipe) on the tortilla, from ½ inch to 1 inch thick, and add finely cut raw salad material such as lettuce, tomatoes, parsley, onions, celery, watercress, avocado, etc.

Sprinkle the tostada with generous amounts of grated cheddar cheese and top with enchilada sauce (see recipe).

VEGETARIAN CHILI NO CARNE

½ c minced parsley
1 c diced celery
½ c cold-pressed oil
1 can tomato sauce
2 garlic cloves, diced

½ tsp chili powder
1 c chopped tomatoes
1 c diced onions
2 c cooked basic kidney
beans (see next recipe)

Saute the onion, and garlic in oil until golden brown. Combine in large saucepan with the beans and remaining ingredients and cook for 10 minutes. Serve with 1 c grated cheddar or Jack cheese.

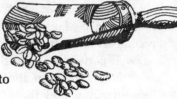

PINTO BEANS

Soak 1 c pinto beans overnight.
Next morning add enough water to
make 1-inch above the beans.

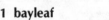

Add to the beans:
1-3 cloves garlic
1 onion, chopped
1 tsp chili powder
1 tbsp Bragg Instant Vegetable Broth Powder

1 bayleaf
1 tbsp Bragg Aminos

Bring the beans to a rolling boil, add seasonings, garlic and onion, and cook for 2 hours or until beans are tender. Then mash the beans and add ¼ pound of natural Jack cheese, grated. Stir well and slowly saute in vegetable oil.

Serve the beans with the enchiladas and the salad. This makes a perfect Mexican meal, topped off with sliced pineapple, either fresh or canned, unsweetened.

LA CASA DIA

On one side of a tortilla place a slice of natural cheddar cheese or Jack cheese (avoid processed cheese). Fold the tortilla in half.

Lightly brush large skillet with oil and over low heat continue turning folded tortilla with spatula until cheese inside is slightly melted and the tortilla is warm.

La Casa Dia can be picked up and eaten as a sandwich.

TACOS

Taco filling:

1 tomato, chopped	⅓ c celery, chopped
½ c lettuce, chopped	¼ c parsley, chopped
¼ c alfalfa sprouts	
⅓ c finely chopped green Bell peppers	
½ c finely chopped avocados (optional)	
Finely chopped onions, either green or dry	

Lay a corn tortilla (heat in pie tin with oil in oven) on a warm plate and spread on parts of each ingredients. We place ingredients on wax paper and let our guests prepare their own tacos. Some might want more onion or none at all, etc. You can vary this by adding more raw grated vegetables. (The sauce must be hot from the stove and guests dip over taco as much sauce as desired.) Try even homemade sauerkraut as a topping.

After folding the taco in half, spoon on enchilada sauce to taste (see recipe for enchilada sauce). The taco can be picked up and eaten, the same as a sandwich.

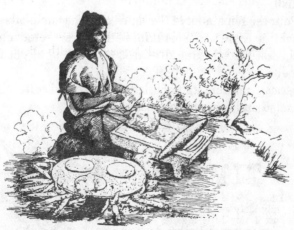

Mexican Woman Making Tortillas

69

ENCHILADAS

First you make an enchilada sauce.
It is very simple to prepare:

3 tbsp chili powder
1 small can tomato sauce   2 c water
3 tbsp cold-pressed soy, safflower or corn oil
1 tbsp yellow or white cornmeal

Brown cornmeal slightly in oil. Add the rest of the ingredients and cook for 10 minutes, stirring constantly to avoid lumps (this is enough sauce for 12 cheese enchiladas).

1. When sauce is done, dip the tortilla in the sauce, then remove it and place on a plate. Continue until all the tortillas have been dipped.

2. Chop very finely 1 cup onions, either green or dry. Grate 2 cups natural cheddar cheese. Remove the tortillas from the plate (one at a time) and spread on the chopped onions and grated cheese. Roll the tortilla and place in baking dish.

3. Pour the remainder of the sauce over the enchiladas in the baking dish and sprinkle with more grated cheddar cheese. Place baking dish in 300° oven until cheese has melted.

(In Mexican restaurants enchiladas are served with a tossed green salad and refried pinto beans.)

TIME

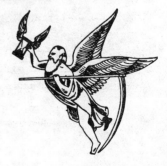

I have just a little minute,
Only sixty seconds in it,
Just a tiny little minute,
Give account if I abuse it;
Forced upon me; can't refuse it.
Didn't seek it, didn't choose it,
But it's up to me to use it.
I must suffer if I lose it;
But eternity is in it.—Unknown.

TAMALE PIE

1 c	cornmeal, natural	1 c	ripe olives, pitted and sliced
2 tbsp	soy oil	¼ c	bell pepper, chopped
¾ c	boiling water	1 tsp	kelp
1 c	garbanzos, soaked	1 tsp	Bragg Aminos
½ c	water	¼ tsp	oregano
1 c	corn, whole kernel	½ tsp	sweet basil
1¾ c	tomatoes, diced	2	garlic clove, pressed
½ c	onions, sauteed		

Pour boiling water over cornmeal and mix thoroughly. Put garbanzos with ½ cup water in blender and chop fine then add to the cornmeal mixture. Reserve sliced olives and two tablespoons of chopped pepper then mix all other ingredients well. Grease a flat baking dish. Pour in ingredients then decorate top with olive slices and chopped pepper. Cover and bake in 375° oven for 25 minutes. Remove lid and bake 20 minutes longer or until firm and well done.

FRIJOLES REFRITOS

½ lb	pinto or red kidney beans	1	onion, sliced
	Water	6 tbsp	soy oil
½ tsp	Italian herbs	½ c	shredded Jack or Cheddar cheese
2 tsp	Bragg Aminos	3	cloves garlic, chopped

Cover beans generously with water and soak overnight. Add Bragg Aminos, sliced onion, garlic and herbs. Cook until beans are very tender, adding more water if needed, but beans should not be soupy. Drain beans of any excess liquid and save for soups or sauces. Heat 3 tablespoons of the oil in a large skillet. Add beans and cook, stirring and mashing with back of spoon to make a paste. Gradually work in remaining oil. Sprinkle with cheese. This is a Bragg favorite, served with a big health salad first—then this bean dish. You can substitute any beans from soya beans to lima beans, they all are delicious.

Ruts long traveled—grow comfortable.

THE HISTORY OF CORN

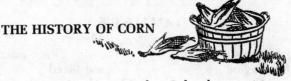

It was on November 5, 1492, that Columbus sent two of his sailors on an exploration trip into the interior of Cuba. They returned to report and brought back with them a grain which the natives called "maize" which had a delicious taste.

On Columbus' return to Europe, the cultivation and use of what was then called Indian corn spread rapidly over the then known world. Within one single generation it became a European food staple. And in two generations it spread into Tibet, India and Africa.

When European ships first arrived in China, they found that corn had preceded them—and that already it was being taxed by the emperor.

Fresh ground cornmeal, either white or yellow, has 41.7% protein in every edible pound of corn. It is rich in calcium, phosphorous, potassium, Vitamin A and natural unsaturated oil.

In Mexico where corn is the grain used for bread, they make a delicious pancake bread called tortillas (tor-tee-yah's), which accompany every meal. Historically, tortillas were made exclusively with cornmeal; this is the reason tortillas are an important part of the Mexican diet from a nutritional standpoint. But I'm very sad to say that both in Mexico and Mexican restaurants in the USA, the tortillas are now made from white flour. These white flour tortillas are tasteless and their nutritional value is close to zero.

When you are buying ready-made tortillas, be absolutely certain that you are buying tortillas made of corn and not tortillas made of white flour. If you cannot purchase corn tortillas at your supermarket, there is a firm in New Mexico that sells tortilla flour and gives excellent recipes on the boxes for making the tortillas. The firm is:

Casados Farms, Box 49, San Juan Pueblo, New Mexico 87566

Please send a self-addressed stamped envelope to obtain the list of products and the prices charged.

SOYBEANS

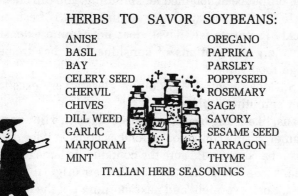

HERBS TO SAVOR SOYBEANS:

ANISE	OREGANO
BASIL	PAPRIKA
BAY	PARSLEY
CELERY SEED	POPPYSEED
CHERVIL	ROSEMARY
CHIVES	SAGE
DILL WEED	SAVORY
GARLIC	SESAME SEED
MARJORAM	TARRAGON
MINT	THYME

ITALIAN HERB SEASONINGS

SOYBEANS

The soybean is one of the richest of all foods in protein and in minerals, and it also makes a very delightful addition to good meals. It has an ancient heritage, having been used for thousands of years by the people of the Orient, but only in recent years have Americans and Europeans become awakened to its possibilities as a meat substitute and also to its great value as a food staple.

HOW TO MAKE SOYBEAN SPROUTS

The sprouts of the soybean do not rightfully belong under the "Beans" classification. They are used as a salad vegetable, to replace salad greens, and can be eaten either cooked or raw. They are a wonderful addition to omelets and meat dishes of all kinds and are, of course, popular in Chinese cookery, as well as in the American adaptation of Chinese cookery such as chow mein, chop suey, and the like.

Bean sprouts can be obtained either from soybeans, mung beans, and other listed beans, and are equally delicious and nutritious. The sprouts can easily be made at home, and their preparation is not difficult.

It is very important to have the finest-quality bean for sprouting. These beans can usually be found at your health food store. They should not be over a year old.

With the proper bean obtained for sprouting, you can create a vegetable in any climate, winter or summer, that is fresh, matures quickly (within a few days), does not require extensive soil cultivation or variations of sunshine, and has tremendously high food value.

The U. S. Department of Agriculture gives a very excellent method for sprouting soybeans:

"Soybeans, like mung beans, can be sprouted in a flower pot, a sink strainer, or any container which has holes in it for drainage, and can be covered. Be sure the container is large enough, for the beans swell to at least six times their original bulk as they sprout. Soak overnight and next morning put the beans in the container, cover, and leave them in a warm place. Flood with lukewarm water at least four or five times each day during the sprouting period. In two to four days, the sprouts will be two to three inches long. Then they should be kept in a cool place, just like any fresh vegetable.

"The sprouts are very tender, and to hold their crispness, should not be added to hot mixtures until a few minutes before serving."

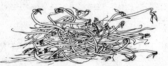

SPROUT SEEDS, BEANS AND GRAINS FOR MORE PROTEIN

Learn to sprout seeds, beans and grains to reap more protein, vitamins, minerals, amino acids and live enzymes compared to their dry state.

ALFALFA SEEDS	GARBANZO BEANS
LENTILS	MUNG BEANS
NAVY BEANS	PINTO BEANS
SOYBEANS	
WHEAT, TRITICALE WHEAT, and other GRAINS	

Let food be your medicine, and medicine be your food.

—Hippocrates

74

SOYBEAN RECIPES

There are so many variations of preparing the magic soybean that we can only give a basic preparation for each type.

GREEN SOYBEANS

Allow soybean pods to stand 10 minutes in boiling water. Drain and shell the beans.

For each cup of the shelled beans, add ½ cup of boiling water. Bring to a boil and cook until beans are tender (10 to 15 minutes). Drain and season in any manner desired.

HOW TO COOK DRIED SOYBEANS

2 c (1 pound) dried soybeans, green or yellow
1 tbsp Bragg Aminos

1. Wash beans well and place in a bowl with water to cover. Soak for 24 hours. As the beans expand up to three times their bulk on soaking, make sure that the bowl is large enough and the water level is 2 or 3 inches above the beans.
2. To cook the beans, place in a heavy kettle with soaking water and extra water, if necessary, to almost cover. Add Bragg Aminos, bring to boil and simmer over low heat 3 or 4 hours or until tender.

   Soybeans will not cook into a soft, mushy mass. They will remain firmer and hold their shape better than the ordinary dry beans.

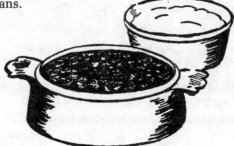

METHOD FOR COOKING BEANS

Wash beans with cold water and remove culls. Ratio is 1 part beans to 3 parts water. Soak overnight and next morning skim off any foam that may have formed. Boil existing water left, add beans to boiling water in heavy pot. Bring to full boil. Turn off heat. Skim again and remove any foam which has formed, then add herbs, garlic and any seasoning desired. There seems to be less flatulence (gas) when beans are cooked and skimmed in this manner.

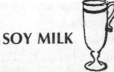

SOY MILK

Soy milk is a liquid resembling cow's milk that can be made from soybeans. It can be used in any recipe calling for ordinary milk and in the same proportions as cow's milk.

There are many ways of making soy milk. This is one of the simplest and most practical and workable recipes: Soak the beans overnight. Measure out three times the amount of liquid in proportion to the soaked beans you have prepared; then grind the beans, adding some of this liquid as you go along, proportioning the liquid so that all of it is used up by the time you have ground all the beans.

Take this pulpy mass and boil it slowly for 1 hour. Strain through a cloth.

If desired, honey, or other sweetening as well as seasoning can be added to taste.

SOYBEAN CHEESE

To prepare soybean cheese, allow soy milk to curdle, just as you would ordinary milk. Set the soy milk in a warm place, and when it is soured and thickened, cut into sections and bring to a boil in a saucepan. Then strain through cloth. The remaining cheese can be seasoned with Bragg Liquid Aminos, onions, chopped chives, or other forms of seasoning.

SOYBEAN CASSEROLE

4 c soybean	3 tbsp dry bread crumbs
1 c chopped celery	2½ tbsp molasses
½ c chopped onions	3 tbsp honey
½ c chopped carrots	2 tbsp olive oil
1 green pepper	2 tbsp parsley, chopped
2½ c fresh tomatoes	1½ tbsp fresh grated ginger (or dry)
1 c raw walnuts (chopped)	grated whole pepper
1 can tomato sauce	2 garlic cloves
6 fresh mushrooms (sauteed)	

Soak soybeans overnight and cook for 30 minutes. Add all other ingredients and mix well. Bake in oiled casserole dish in 350° oven for 45 minutes.

SOYBEAN AND VEGETABLE STEW

4 potatoes, sliced	4 large tomatoes, sliced
2 large onions, sliced	1 tbsp Bragg Aminos
2 celery stalks, diced	½ tsp Italian herbs
1 green pepper, sliced	dash of cayenne
4 tbsp soy oil	2½ c soybeans, cooked

Place soy oil in heavy skillet then add potatoes (skins too), onions, celery, green pepper. Sprinkle Bragg aminos and cayenne over vegetables then add beans and tomatoes. Cover and cook very slowly about an hour or until done, adding liquid from soybeans or water if needed.

SAUTEED SOYBEAN SPROUTS AND ONIONS

1 lb soybean sprouts	2 to 4 tbsp Bragg Aminos
4 tbsp soy oil	1½ tbsp cornstarch
3 onions, chopped	4 tbsp water
1 c vegetable stock	

Lightly saute sprouts and onions in soy oil. Add vegetable stock and Bragg Aminos. Thicken with cornstarch and water made into a paste and serve hot.

BOSTON BAKED SOYBEANS

2½ c canned or fresh cooked
    soybeans
½ tsp mustard
2 tbsp unsulphured
    molasses

¼ minced onion
3 tbsp soy oil
¼ tsp ground fresh
    peppercorns
2 garlic cloves, crushed

Mix all ingredients together. Bake in a buttered casserole in a moderate oven 350° 20 to 30 minutes. Serves 5.

STUFFED PEPPERS WITH SOYBEANS

4 green peppers
¼ c diced cucumber
1 c canned or fresh cooked
    soybeans
¼ minced onion

¼ c diced celery
2 ripe tomatoes
1 tsp minced chives
¼ tsp thyme

Remove seeds from green pepper by cutting off top near the stem and hollowing out. Boil very slowly for 5 minutes. Mash soybeans. Cook celery and cucumber until almost tender. Peel and section tomatoes, cut into fine pieces. Make a mixture of the beans, vegetables, and seasoning. Stuff peppers; cover top with a few whole-wheat buttered bread crumbs. Bake in hot oven for about 20 to 25 minutes. Serves 4.

SOYBEAN SPROUTS EN CASSEROLE

3 c sprouted soybeans
3 sliced onions
¾ c celery
½ c whole-wheat bread
    crumbs

1 c milk
2 tbsp soybean flour
¾ c grated cheese
2 egg yolks
3 tbsp butter or peanut oil

Lightly sauté sprouts, onions, and celery. Add this to beaten egg yolk, milk, and seasoning. Put mixture into buttered casserole. Top with grated cheese and bread crumbs. Bake in a moderate oven for 25 to 30 minutes, or until delicately brown. Serves 6.

SOYBEAN-RICE LOAF

2 c soybeans,
  cooked & chopped
1 c brown rice, cooked
2 eggs, unbeaten
2 tbsp tomato sauce

3 tbsp onion, minced
2 garlic cloves, minced
1 tbsp lemon juice
½ tsp celery seed
1 tsp Bragg Aminos

Mix ingredients in order given. Put in greased loaf pan and Bake 350° oven for 20 minutes. Sprinkle with grated cheese last 5 minutes if desired.

BAKED SOYBEAN CROQUETTES

2 tbsp onion, minced
1 garlic, minced
1½ c celery, diced
1½ tsp Bragg Aminos
1 c tomato puree
2 tbsp soy oil

5 tbsp whole wheat
  flour
3 c soybean pulp
  Wheat germ, raw
1 egg, well beaten
2 tbsp water

Add minced onion, garlic, celery, and Bragg Aminos to tomato puree and bring to a boil. Mix flour and oil together and add the boiling tomato puree mixture slowly. Cook to a thick paste. Cool and add soybean pulp. Soybean pulp is prepared by pressing cooked soybeans through a coarse sieve or by grinding them in a food grinder, or blender. Shape into croquettes. Roll in wheat germ, then in beaten egg to which water has been added, and again in wheat germ. Place on a greased baking sheet and bake in a 400° oven for 20 to 30 minutes.

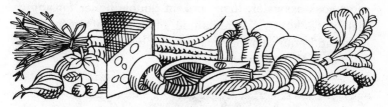

What sculpture is to a block of marble, education is to the soul.
—Addison, The Spectator

SOYBEAN PATTIES WITH TOMATO SAUCE

1 c soybeans, soaked	1 tbsp soy oil
½ c water	¼ tsp onion powder
2 tbsp flake yeast or	speck of garlic powder
tbsp powdered yeast	1 tsp Italian herbs
1 tbsp Bragg Aminos	⅝ c rolled oats

Grind soybeans in food chopper and then combine with the remainder of the ingredients. If you prefer, you may combine all the ingredients, with the exception of the rolled oats, and chop fine in blender — then add the oats. Regardless of which method you use, all ingredients should be left standing for 10 minutes to absorb all moisture. Drop mixture in mounds equalling approximately ½ cup on baking pan which has been well oiled. Bake in 350° oven for 10 minutes or until nicely browned. Turn and cover then bake 10 more minutes. Reduce heat to 325° and cook an additional 10 minutes. Serve with a tomato sauce which can be prepared as follows:

SOYBEAN LOAF

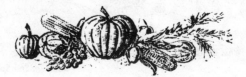

2 c soy beans	1 onion, chopped
1 c wholewheat bread crumbs	1 bunch spinach, chopped
	½ tsp Italian herbs
¼ c uncooked wholewheat cereal	2 tbsp soy or olive oil
	2 garlic cloves, mashed
1 c raw carrots, chop finely	1 tsp Bragg Aminos

Soak beans overnight, skim off foam and grind. Cover with same soaking water, then cook in double boiler for approximately two hours. Add remainder of ingredients to cooked soy beans and pour in a loaf or ring pan. Bake 30 minutes in 350° oven or until lightly browned.

SOYBEAN STUFFED PEPPERS

8-9 green peppers
1 tsp Bragg Aminos
2 c Soybean pulp
1 tsp onions, minced
½ c celery, diced

½ c fresh tomatoes, chopped
whole wheat bread crumbs
1 tsp kelp seasoning

Remove seeds and inner partitions from green peppers. Parboil peppers for 3 minutes. At same time simmer celery in another pan containing ¼ cup of water. Sprinkle inside of peppers with kelp seasoning. Fill with mixture of bean pulp, celery, tomatoes, onion and aminos. Cover tops with whole wheat bread crumbs. Place in greased pan and bake in 400° oven for 30 minutes or until the peppers are soft.

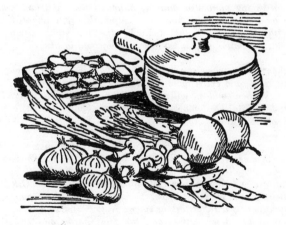

Surely if living creatures saw the consequences of all their evil deeds, with hatred would they turn and leave them, fearing the ruin following.
—F'shuing Tsan K'ung

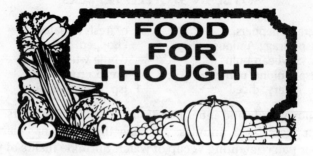

FOOD FOR THOUGHT

Now good digestion waits on appetite, and health on both. — Shakespeare

We live not upon what we eat, but upon what we digest. — Abernethy

Almost every human malady is connected, either by highway or byway, with the stomach. — Sir Francis Head

It is a well-established fact that a leg of mutton caused a revolution in the affairs of Europe. Just before the battle of Leipsic, Napoleon the Great insisted on dining on boiled mutton, although his physicians warned him that it would disagree with him. The emperor's brain resented the liberty taken with its colleague, the stomach; the monarch's equilibrium was overturned, the battle lost, and a new page opened in history.

The kitchen [that is, your stomach] being out of order, the garret [the head] cannot be right, and every room in the house becomes affected. Remedy the evil in the kitchen, and all will be right in parlor and chamber. If you put improper food into the stomach, you play the mischief with it, and with the whole machine besides. — Abernethy

Cattle know when to go home from grazing, but a foolish man never knows his stomach's measures. — Scandinavian Proberb

Simplicity of diet is the characteristic of the dwellers in the Orient. According to Niebuhr, the sheik of the desert wants only a dish of pillau, or boiled rice, which he eats without fork or spoon. Notwithstanding their frugal fare, these sons of the desert are among the most hardy and enduring of all members of the human family. A traveler tells of seeing one of them run up to the top of the tallest pyramid and back in six minutes.

One fourth of what we eat keeps us, and the other three fourths we keep at the peril of our lives. — Abernethy

Bad cooking diminishes happiness and shortens life. — Wisdom of Ages

Says Mrs. Partington: "Many a fair home has been desiccated by poor cooking, and a man's table has been the rock on which his happiness has split."

APPETIZERS

"APPETIZERS" are a misnomer and, contrary to popular belief, do not point up the appetite but rather dull it. The very best appetizer for a meal is a small glass of fruit or vegetable juice or a good crisp salad. But for a gala occasion the so-called appetizers, or canapés, are nice to serve with fruit or vegetable juice cocktails, and they can be prepared the Health way.

Appetizers should never be substantial. They should be spicy tidbits and of distinctive flavor to pique the activity of the gastric juices. If they are to be served just prior to a meal, the soup course of the meal should be omitted. Ordinarily, the appetizers contain good proportions of fatty substances—cheeses, spreads, and oils. Soup, immediately following the appetizers adds additional fatty substances, causing a too rapid and false satisfaction of the appetite.

Delicious appetizers can be made without the usual smoked, pickled, or processed meats or fish. Most of the canapé tidbits to follow may be served on small, thin squares of dry, toasted whole-wheat bread, rye bread, or whole-grain crackers, unless otherwise indicated.

SNAPPY CHEESE BALLS

Use a nippy cheese. Cut into balls or cubes. Roll in mayonnaise, then celery or mustard seed. Place one small leaf of watercress or mint on top of each ball or cube and stab into place with toothpick.

KNOBBY CHEESE BALLS

Make round balls of cream cheese and avocado can be added if desired. Blend with green pepper and watercress, chopped fine. Form into small balls about the size of butter balls. Roll in poppy seed, insert toothpick in each one, and serve on bed of parsley or watercress.

STUFFED CELERY

2 tbsp Roquefort cheese   **2 tbsp cottage cheese**

Mash, blend thoroughly. Spread mixture on inside of celery stalk. Sprinkle top of cheese with celery seed, caraway seed, sesame seed, or anise. (Do not combine these seeds; use only one for your flavoring.)

VARIATIONS FOR STUFFED CELERY

1. Peanut butter.
2. Mashed avocado blended with 1 teaspoon minced chives and ⅛ tsp (or less) thyme.
3. Any unprocessed cheese blended with chives, chervil, thyme, or marjoram.
4. Cream cheese blended with minced onion or chives.

AVOCADO PASTE

Mash avocado. Cream with celery, green bell pepper, chives or bits of onion chopped fine. Sprinkle with sesame seeds or caraway.

84

CELERY STICKS

Wash and dry thoroughly stalks of celery. Cut in 4 inch lengths.

Mash yogurt and cottage cheese together and then fill in the grooves of the celery stalk.

Blue cheese may be added to this mixture for a more tasty celery stick.

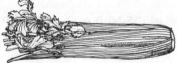

SPROUTS-BEANS APPETIZER

3 c alfalfa, mung and lentil sprouts, Sprouted in combination
1 lb fresh or canned wax beans cooked, drained
1 lb fresh or canned green beans cooked, drained

1 lb kidney beans or garbanzos cooked, drained
½ c apply cider vinegar
½ c olive oil
⅓ c Honey
1 tbsp Bragg Aminos
3 cloves of garlic, minced
1 c Onion, chopped

Put sprouts and beans in bowl. Mix remaining ingredients and puree in blender. Pour over beans and sprouts, toss well, cover and marinate in refrigerator overnight.

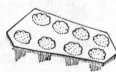

CHEESE PUFFS

1 lb cheddar cheese
½ tsp ground mustard
1 tbsp cellu baking powder

4 tbsp melted butter, salt-free
4 egg whites, beaten stiff

Cellu health baking powder is available at health food stores.

Grate cheese fine, add all other ingredients, and stir; add whites of eggs last. Put on small wafers or rounds of toast. Toast under broiler before serving, and serve while hot. Serves 10.

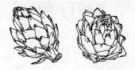

ARTICHOKE HEARTS

Stuff artichoke hearts with a mixture of nippy cheese and bread crumbs, blended. Sprinkle with celery, poppy, or mustard seed. Place under broiler for a few moments and brown. Cut in quarters, stab with toothpick, serve on nasturtium leaves.

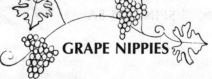

GRAPE NIPPIES

Select large, firm green grapes. Slit, remove seeds. Fill center with mixture of ¾ cream cheese to ¼ Roquefort cheese, with a few drops of lemon juice for blending. Remove excess paste around edges. Pierce through with long toothpick. Chill before serving.

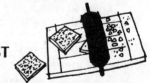

HERB TOAST

½ c melted butter
¼ tsp of each of the following: chives, basil, marjoram, thyme

Allow herbs to stand in butter for 30 minutes. Reheat butter. Saturate several slices whole-wheat bread. Place in oven to brown, and toast slowly for about 20 to 25 minutes. Remove, cut in small pieces and serve.

MUSHROOMS

Broil mushrooms covered with butter and roll in chopped chives. Stab with toothpick.

SALADS AND DRESSINGS

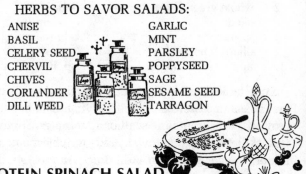

HERBS TO SAVOR SALADS:

ANISE	GARLIC
BASIL	MINT
CELERY SEED	PARSLEY
CHERVIL	POPPYSEED
CHIVES	SAGE
CORIANDER	SESAME SEED
DILL WEED	TARRAGON

HI-PROTEIN SPINACH SALAD

1 bunch (or more) fresh
  raw green spinach
2 hard-boiled eggs

1 c sliced raw mushrooms
Fresh thinly sliced onions
to taste.

THE DRESSING FOR THIS SALAD:

A mixture of natural apple cider vinegar, fresh lemon juice, oil and honey. Combine this to taste.

LENTIL TOSTADA SALAD

2 c lettuce, chopped
⅓ c celery, chopped
⅓ c green onions, chopped
⅓ c cucumbers, sliced
¼ c parsley, chopped
6 tomatoes, diced
6 whole wheat toast slices or corn tortilla, heated

3 c lentils, cooked
½ c health salad dressing
½ c soy cream
1 tbs lemon juice
⅛ tsp garlic powder
¼ tsp kelp seasoning

Mix together lettuce, green onions, celery, parsley and cucumbers and set to one side. Put salad dressing in bowl. Add lemon juice and garlic powder, and mix well. Set to one side. Toast bread or heat tortillas. Spread with salad dressing. Spoon hot lentils on top of toast. Cover with chopped salad greens. Top with diced tomato. Drizzle salad dressing over all. Eat with fork.

HOT SPROUT SALAD

3 tbsp soy oil	1 tsp whole wheat
2 c whole green beans, cooked	flour
	¼ c warm water
2 c sprouts	kelp seasoning
2 scallions, chopped	(to taste)
½ c apple cider vinegar	1 tsp Bragg Aminos

In one tablespoon of soy oil, heat drained beans two minutes. Place beans in casserole or other serving dish. In one tablespoon of soy oil, heat sprouts and scallions 2 minutes. Stir into casserole. Clean skillet with paper towel. Add one tablespoon oil. Heat. Stir in flour, vinegar and water. Add Bragg Aminos, stir until boiling. Pour sauce over sprouts and beans. Sprinkle with kelp seasoning if desired. Keep warm until ready to serve.

ITALIAN HERB SEASONING*

1 tsp thyme	1 tbsp rosemary
1 tsp paprika	2 tbsp oregano
2 tbsp basil	1 tsp tarragon
1 tsp garlic powder (optional)	

Place all ingredients in an air-tight container. Cover and shake thoroughly to blend.
Yield: Approximately ½ cup.

*You can purchase an Italian seasoning at your grocery's spice dept. but, we prefer to make our own and the more you use herbs, the greater delight in flavors you will discover. In the Bragg garden we always have an herb section, then you can dry and store them and mix your own for recipes as needed.

The above combination is delicious in most all vegetarian recipes—you try it and can vary it to your taste as you learn what herbs appeal most to you. You may wish to add garlic powder to say half of the mixture and make up two small jars: Italian Herb Seasoning and Italian Herb & Garlic Seasoning.

VEGETARIAN RECIPES FROM THE "LONGER LIFE, HEALTH AND HAPPINESS CLUB"

Every morning, Monday through Saturday, on the beautiful Fort DeRussy officers' compound at Waikiki Beach, Hawaii, a group of health minded people meet with me for deep breathing, exercising, meditation, group singing and mini-lectures on how to live a long, healthy life. Membership in the club is free and open to everyone.

On Sundays a group from the club travels to one of the most beautiful spots on the island of Oahu, known as Waimea Bay Park. This is called our "health day" and we start our program by walking and jogging on the beautiful green lawn of the park. We then walk up to what we have named "Breathatarian Hill" which is a high promontory that affords a magnificent view of the beautiful north side of Oahu Island.

There is a fresh water river that comes down from the Waimea Falls in which we spend happy times swimming and enjoying the fresh, crystal clear water. We call this river "the River of Life" because we actually feel that its sparkling, rejuvenating water increases our life force.

We then go to the ocean to swim at one of the best beaches in these beautiful islands.

At 12:00 noon we all sit down to a potluck health luncheon. Our members have come up with some extraordinary recipes which are great favorites of the group, and we are sharing some of them with you.

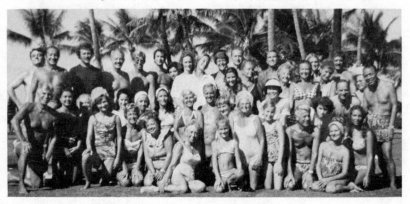

BEETS DELIGHT
Connie Godlove's

6 or 8 beets—cooked, peeled and sliced.
Saute 2 cloves crushed garlic in ½ c olive oil, ½ c vinegar, 2 tbsp honey ½ c orange juice 1½ tsp grated orange peel and 1 c juice off the beets.
Place beets in this hot sauce and add a large sliced onion, 5 pepper corns, 1 bayleaf, parsley, fresh herbs (basil, tarragon, marjoram, rosemary).
Marinate 48 hours or more.

GREEN BEAN-ONION SALAD
Fred and Jean Pump's

1 pound fresh green beans, sliced, cooked	2 tbsp natural cider vinegar
⅓ c olive oil	¼ tsp crushed dried basil
1 c finely chopped onions, either dry or green, using stems	

Mix all ingredients and marinate. Chill one hour and serve.

STRING BEAN SALAD OR GARNISH

2 c string beans sliced	1 c thin strips of Swiss cheese
½ c onion finely chopped	
1 tbsp Bragg Aminos	1 tbsp honey
¼ tsp dry mustard	3 tbsp olive oil
pinch Basil powder	2 tbsp Apple cider vinegar

Cook the string beans and sprinkle over them, the onion and honey. Mix well. Cover tightly and chill.

In a small jar shake together the oil, vinegar, basil, Bragg Aminos and mustard. Set aside. When serving, turn the beans into a salad bowl and add oil mixture and toss well. Add the cheese over the top. This can be a garnish for other salads.

Men do not die, they KILL themselves. —Seneca, Roman Philosopher

GREEN PEPPER STUFFED WITH COTTAGE CHEESE

Cut green pepper in half. Remove seeds. Fill with cottage cheese and top with pumpkin seeds.

Cottage cheese has plenty of first class proteins and for a quick meal this can be eaten with chopped vegetables, an apple, a pear, or grapes; in fact, any fruits or vegetables.

FRENCH DRESSING WITH TOMATO JUICE

⅓ c lemon juice
⅓ c soy oil
1½ tbsp honey
1 tbsp Bragg Aminos

1 c tomato juice
1 garlic clove, crushed
½ tsp sweet basil
½ tsp rosemary

Blend well; allow to stand. Will make 1⅓ cups.

GRAPEFRUIT FRENCH DRESSING

4 tbsp olive oil
1 tbsp grapefruit juice
½ tbsp lemon juice

¼ tsp paprika
1 tbsp finely crumbled
Roquefort cheese

Blend ingredients, beat vigorously. Allow to stand one hour before serving. Will make ¼ cup.

TOMATO SAUCE

2 c tomatoes, cooked
½ c onions, finely chopped, sauteed
½ c green pepper, chopped
1 c tomatoes, finely chopped

1 tbsp soy oil
1 tbsp honey
½ tsp Bragg Aminos
1 tsp sweet basil
1 garlic clove, crushed

Place juice from 2 cups cooked tomatoes in sauce pan with sauteed onions and chopped pepper. Bring to boil and let simmer until volume is reduced by half, then add 1 cup of tomatoes in small pieces and add to juice together with the seasoning. Let simmer briefly or until mixture is quite thick.

HONEY CELERY SEED DRESSING

1 tsp dry mustard	1 medium onion, grated
1 tsp Bragg Aminos	⅓ c apple cider vinegar
¼ tsp paprika	1 c soy oil
⅓ c honey	1 tbsp celery seed

Measure dry ingredients into small mixing bowl, then add honey and Bragg Aminos and thoroughly blend. Add grated onion and small amount of the apple cider vinegar. Beat mixture. Add oil and remaining apple cider vinegar alternately. Celery seed should be added last. Store in a cool place in covered jar. Makes approximately 2 cups.

HONEY FRENCH DRESSING

⅔ c olive or soy oil	6 tbsp lemon juice
½ c honey	1 tsp kelp seasoning

Mix all ingredients except honey. Add honey slowly and beat vigorously. Will make 1½ cups.

HONEY SOY-OIL DRESSING

¼ med. onion, grated	5½ tbsp lemon juice
1 c soy oil	3 tsp celery seed
1 tsp dry mustard	½ tsp paprika
½ c orange-blossom honey	

Measure dry ingredients into small mixing bowl. Add honey and blend thoroughly. Add grated onion and small amount of lemon juice. Beat mixture; add oil and remaining lemon juice alternately and then celery seed. Store in a covered jar in a cool place. Will make 1½ cups.

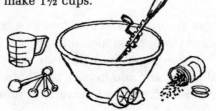

ROQUEFORT DRESSING

½ lb Roquefort cheese   lemon juice
  olive, soy, or peanut oil

Mash Roquefort cheese with fork adding lemon juice to give the cheese a thick yet smooth consistency; add enough oil so that it is smooth. Will make 1 cup.

LEMON MAYONNAISE

2 c soy, peanut, or olive oil   1 tsp dry mustard
½ c lemon juice   2 egg yolks
¼ tsp thyme

Combine dry ingredients with unbeaten yolks in a mixing bowl and beat together until stiff. Add part of the oil, beating it into the mixture drop by drop at first, then proceeding more rapidly, keeping the mixture firm. When it begins to thicken, add a little lemon juice alternately with the oil. Makes 2½ cups.

RUSSIAN DRESSING

½ c lemon mayonnaise   1 tbsp chopped pimiento
¼ c chili sauce   ½ tsp anise seed
1 tbsp celery seed   1 garlic clove, crushed
1 tbsp chopped green   ½ tsp honey
  pepper

Blend ingredients; beat vigorously and allow to stand for one hour before serving. Will make ¾ cup.

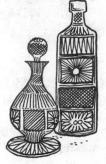

DILL-SEED DRESSING

½ tsp dry mustard
1 tsp honey
¾ tbsp lemon juice
¼ c whipped cream

1 hard-boiled egg yolk
1 uncooked egg yolk
½ c olive, soy, or peanut oil
½ tsp dill seed

Rub cooked egg yolk through a sieve, add uncooked egg yolk. Beat in oil gradually, add lemon juice and seasonings. Just before serving fold in whipped cream and dill seed. Makes 1 cup.

SOUR-CREAM DRESSING

1 c sour cream
2 hard-boiled egg yolks

½ tsp orange-blossom honey
1 tsp lemon juice

Press yolks through a sieve and beat into sour cream. Beat in lemon juice, honey. Makes 1¼ cups.

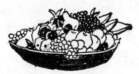

QUICK SOUR-CREAM DRESSING
FOR VEGETABLE SALADS

To one cup thick sour cream add the juice of one half to one lemon. Mix well and serve with desired salad. This is excellent for cooked vegetables. Add seasonings as desired.

QUICK SOUR-CREAM DRESSING
FOR FRUIT SALADS

To the above recipe, substitute orange or pineapple juice in place of lemon. Add a small amount of honey if desired.

FRENCH SOUR-CREAM DRESSING

Thin thick sour cream with a small amount of French tomato dressing. For variation minced chives, ripe olives, watercress, or minced cucumbers may be added.

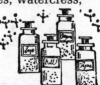

INDIAN SALAD DRESSING

1 tbsp minced green pepper
1 tbsp minced red pepper
1 tbsp minced cooked beets
2 tsp minced parsley
¼ tsp paprika
1 tbsp grapefruit or lemon
    juice, fresh

½ tsp orange-blossom honey
2 hard-boiled egg yolks
½ c olive, soy, or peanut oil
2 tbsp lemon juice
¼ tsp thyme

Press the egg yolks through a sieve; combine all ingredients. Toss until well blended. Good with avocado salads and vegetable salads. Makes about 1 cup.

MUSTARD DRESSING

⅓ c lemon juice
⅔ c olive oil
1 tbsp honey

1 tsp mustard seed
1 tsp peppercorn freshly
    ground

Blend all ingredients and allow to stand one hour before serving. Will make 1 cup.

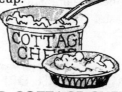

AVOCADO AND COTTAGE CHEESE DRESSING

2 mashed avocados
1 c cottage cheese

juice of 1 lemon

Mix mashed avocados and cottage cheese thoroughly, add the juice of lemon. Beat to a creamy consistency. Add seasoning as desired. Will make 2 cups.

LIME DRESSING

4 tbsp olive oil
2 tbsp fresh lime juice
1 tsp oregano

1 tsp celery seed
1 tsp honey

Blend ingredients, beat vigorously. Allow to stand for one hour before serving. Makes ¼ cup.

FRUIT-SALAD COOKED DRESSING

1½ c sour cream
6 egg yolks
¼ c lemon juice

2 tsps honey
½ tsp mint, crushed
¼ c orange juice, fresh

Beat egg yolks until creamy. Add sour cream slowly while beating. Blend in other ingredients; mix thoroughly. Cook in a double boiler until it thickens, stirring constantly. Remove immediately as mixture begins to thicken, to prevent curdling. Makes 3 cups.

PINEAPPLE-DELIGHT DRESSING

2 pkgs cream cheese
orange-blossom honey

pineapple juice

Mash cream cheese. Add enough pineapple juice to give the consistency of whipped cream. Add enough honey to sweeten for your particular taste. This is a delicious fruit-salad dressing. Makes 1 cup.

TOMATO-JUICE DRESSING

1 c tomato juice
½ c soy oil
3 tbsp lemon juice
2 tsp Bragg Aminos

¾ tsp dry mustard
1 tsp minced onion
1 tsp chives, minced
1 garlic clove, crushed

Mix all ingredients until well blended. Beat thoroughly. Will make 1½ cups.

96

SOUPS IMPORTANT IN A VEGETARIAN DIET

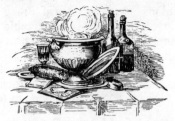

HERBS TO SAVOR SOUPS:

ANISE	OREGANO
BASIL	PARSLEY
BAY	ROSEMARY
CARAWAY	SAGE
CHERVIL	SAVORY
CHIVES	SUMMER
CORIANDER	TARRAGON
DILL WEED	THYME

ITALIAN HERB SEASONINGS

Many delicious and nutritious soups rich in protein can be made such as barley soup, millet soup, mushroom soup, dried lima bean soup, kidney bean soup, pinto bean soup, navy bean soup and lentil soup. Lentil soup is our favorite and supplies a large share of the daily requirement for protein, vitamin and mineral needs. Unlike dried peas and beans, lentils cook quickly (30 minutes) without pre-soaking. Once you become acquainted with the taste of lentil soup, you will rejoice in its hearty deliciousness. Here is the Bragg favorite lentil soup.

BRAGG LENTIL SOUP

1½ c lentils, washed
 1 qt water
 1 tbsp Bragg Aminos
 1 c chopped parsley
 1 c carrots
 1 c chopped onions
 ½ tsp Italian Herb Seasoning

1 c chopped green pepper
1 c chopped celery
3 tomatoes
2 cloves garlic (optional)
1 tsp Bragg Instant
    Vegetable Broth Powder

Combine all ingredients; simmer (covered) 30 minutes or until done.

SPLIT PEA SOUP

1 c split peas
1 c chopped onions
1 c chopped carrots
½ c chopped parsley
¾ c chopped celery
1 bayleaf
½ tsp Italian Herb
   Seasoning

¼ tsp marjoram leaves
1 tsp Bragg Instant
   Vegetable Powder
1 tbsp Bragg Aminos
2 cloves garlic (optional)
1 tbsp unsalted butter or
   cold-pressed oil
½ c cream (optional)

Soak peas overnight in cold water. Do not drain; add all other ingredients and water to cover, and cook until peas are mushy. Just before serving, add the cream and the butter or oil.

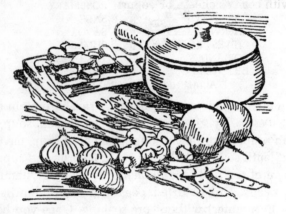

GOLDEN SOUP

1 Spanish sweet onion
½ lb ripe tomatoes
1½ pt vegetable water or
   Bragg Vegetable Broth
1 tbsp Bragg Aminos

3 tbsp soy oil
½ tsp Italian Herbs
½ c Parmesan Cheese,
   grated
2 cloves garlic, sliced

Cook the peeled and sliced onion and garlic in the soy oil until golden. Add the sliced tomatoes and cook for 65 minutes, then add Italian herbs, Bragg Aminos. Simmer very slowly for 15 minutes. Pass soup through a sieve, return to pan and reheat. Put heaping tablespoon of Parmesan Cheese in bowl then ladle soup over it.

ZUCCHINI SOUP

1 pound zucchini (5 small)
washed and sliced
⅛ tsp basil
⅛ tsp thyme
⅛ tsp marjoram
2 c milk
1 c cottage cheese or yogurt
2 tsp Bragg Instant Vegetable Broth Powder

1 c water
1 bayleaf
½ c chopped parsley
1 tbsp Bragg Aminos
1 clove garlic, mashed
(optional)

(1) Place the zucchini, herbs, garlic, and water in (covered) saucepan and simmer gently until tender. (2) Add all the other ingredients. Stir in the milk and heat, but do not boil. (3) Serve topped with cottage cheese or yogurt.

SUNFLOWER SEED SOUP

¾ c grated carrots
1 large onion, finely
chopped
2 tbsp oil or unsalted
butter
1½ c water

1 bayleaf
1 tbsp Bragg Aminos
1 tsp Bragg Instant
Vegetable
Broth Powder
1 tbsp honey

3 medium sized tomatoes (skin and blend in an electric blender until smooth)
½ c sunflower meal (This may be purchased at your health food store or can be made in your blender or in what is called a "grain, nut and seed electric blender" which also can be purchased at your health food store.)

(1) Heat the oil or butter in a saucepan and saute carrots and onions over low heat, about 3 minutes. Add water, cover and cook until vegetables are barely tender. (2) Add vegetable mixture, including the liquid, to the tomato mixture in the blender and blend until smooth. (3) Pour the mixture back into the saucepan and add the Braggs Aminos, Bragg Broth, honey and sunflower meal. Reheat to below simmer point, stirring constantly. (4) To make this more nutritious, when poured into bowl garnish with 1 tbsp. yogurt, chopped green onion (using entire onion and stem) and even avocado slices are delicious.

Take time
for **12** things

1 **Take time to Work—**
   it is the price of success.

2 **Take time to Think—**
   it is the source of power.

3 **Take time to Play—**
   it is the secret of youth.

4 **Take time to Read—**
   it is the foundation of knowledge.

5 **Take time to Worship—**
   it is the highway of reverance and washes the
   dust of earth from our eyes.

6 **Take time to Help and Enjoy Friends—**
   it is the source of happiness.

7 **Take time to Love—**
   it is the one sacrament of life.

8 **Take time to Dream—**
   it hitches the soul to the stars.

9 **Take time to Laugh—**
   it is the singing that helps with life's loads.

10 **Take time for Beauty—**
   it is everywhere in nature.

11 **Take time for Health—**
   it is the true wealth and treasure of life.

12 **Take time to Plan—**
   it is the secret of being able to have time to
   take time for the first eleven things.

VEGETABLES

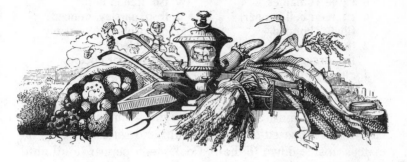

HERBS TO SAVOR VEGETABLES:

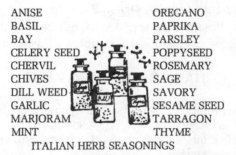

ANISE	OREGANO
BASIL	PAPRIKA
BAY	PARSLEY
CELERY SEED	POPPYSEED
CHERVIL	ROSEMARY
CHIVES	SAGE
DILL WEED	SAVORY
GARLIC	SESAME SEED
MARJORAM	TARRAGON
MINT	THYME

ITALIAN HERB SEASONINGS

RAW AND COOKED VEGETABLES
IMPORTANT TO A MEATLESS DIET

Vegetables as well as fruit, both raw in salads and properly cooked, are among the "protective" foods, and should represent at least three fifths of the diet. These foods not only contribute vitamins and minerals to the diet, but add the bulk required for proper body functioning. In addition to helping maintain the alkaline reserve of the body, they add variety, color, flavor, and texture to the diet.

To a long generation of Americans, vegetables have been a colorless, unappetizing, and uninteresting food, and no wonder. The accustomed method of boiling all the life out of the most succulent garden-picture vegetables and serving them straight from a swimming pool of surplus cooking water is certainly an unappetizing way to serve nature's delicacies.

CORNBREAD STUFFED TOMATOES

6 Large Tomatoes	¼ tsp Italian herbs
¼ c green bell pepper, finely chopped	2 tbsp parsley, minced
2 tbsp soy oil	2½ c Cornbread, coarsely crumbled
1 tsp Bragg Aminos	⅓ c Cheddar cheese, grated (optional)
1 clove garlic, pressed	

Cut a thin slice from stem end of each tomato. Gently spoon out seeds and most of the pulp, leaving firm shells. Chop ½ cup of the squeezed-out tomato pulp and set aside. Turn tomatoes upside down to drain. Cook green pepper in oil until tender but not browned. Add Bragg Aminos, Italian herbs, garlic, parsley, cornbread and chopped tomatoes. Mix lightly. Stuff lightly into tomato shells. Place in a greased shallow baking dish. Bake at 350° for 15 to 20 minutes. Sprinkle grated Cheddar cheese over top last 5 minutes—this is optional.

HAWAIIAN SAUERKRAUT

½ lb sauerkraut	½ c pineapple, fresh, chopped
½ lb red cabbage	1 c tomatoes, chopped
2 tbsp olive oil	
1 tsp Bragg Aminos	

The sauerkraut comes in its own juice which you use for cooking. Shred the red cabbage and simmer all ingredients except oil and aminos together for 30 minutes. Allow to cool, then reheat and add the oil and aminos. Serve very hot.

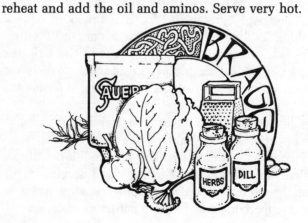

SOYBEAN SPROUTS WITH ONIONS AND MUSHROOMS

3 c sprouted soybeans	4 tbsp Bragg Liquid Aminos
½ c onion tops, chopped fine	1 c mushrooms, sliced
	3 tbsp butter, salt free

Sauté onion tops, bean sprouts, and mushrooms lightly in butter. Pour Aminos over the mixture and allow to simmer for a few moments before serving. Serves 5.

STUFFED BAKED POTATOES

Bake three large russet potatoes. When done, cut in half, scoop out up to ¼ inch of the skin. Place the scooped out portion in a mixing bowl and add:

¼ pound unsalted butter
1 c grated natural cheese
½ c green onions, cut very small (using the green stems)

Mash the mixture, then with a spoon fill it into the half potato shells; sprinkle on paprika. Place in 375° oven for 15 - 20 minutes, allowing the cheese to melt. Serves 6.

BROILED STUFFED SQUASH

4 large Summer Squashes	1 tbsp Bragg Aminos
½ c Blue Cheese, crumbled	1 clove garlic, pressed
	1 tsp soy oil
⅓ c raw wheat germ or fine dry whole wheat crumbs	

Cut off stem ends of squash. Blanch in boiling water for 4 minutes. Drain and scoop out inside leaving shells whole. Add oil and garlic. Combine squash pulp, wheat germ or fine dry whole wheat crumbs with blue cheese. Fill shells with this mixture then place in shallow baking dish and broil 5 minutes to melt cheese.

NUTTED ONION CUPS

6 Onions, large	¼ c parsley, minced
¼ c Soy Oil	2 c dry whole wheat crumbs
¼ c celery, diced	½ c walnuts, chopped
½ tsp rubbed sage	¼ c Parmesan cheese,
1 clove garlic, minced	grated
1 tsp kelp seasoning	1 tbsp Bragg Aminos

Peel onions & cut a thin slice from each end. Using a skewer, pierce each onion several times from top through center to prevent them collapsing while cooking. Stand onions upright in a saucepan in which they fit snugly, cover with boiling water, cover pot and bring to boil. Simmer 30 minutes or until onions are tender but not soft. Cool and scoop out centers. Chop centers and set aside. Meanwhile heat soy oil in skillet. Brush onions with oil. Cook celery and onion in remaining oil until celery is tender. Add sage, garlic, kelp seasoning, parsley and bread crumbs. Mix well and remove from heat. Stir in nuts, cheese and Bragg Liquid Aminos. Spoon mixture into onion cups. Arrange in a greased shallow baking dish and bake in 325° oven for 35 minutes.

HONEY CARROT PUDDING

1 c carrots, grated	1 egg
1 c raisins	1 tbsp cinnamon
½ c honey	1 c whole wheat flour
1 c grated potatoes,	⅓ c soy oil
skin too	½ tsp kelp granules

Mix well, and steam for 1½-2 hours in double boiler or in oven. Serve piping hot. Top with yogurt or kefir if desired when served.

CASEROLES

HERBS TO SAVOR CASSEROLES:

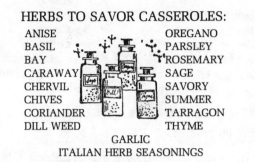

ANISE	OREGANO
BASIL	PARSLEY
BAY	ROSEMARY
CARAWAY	SAGE
CHERVIL	SAVORY
CHIVES	SUMMER
CORIANDER	TARRAGON
DILL WEED	THYME

GARLIC
ITALIAN HERB SEASONINGS

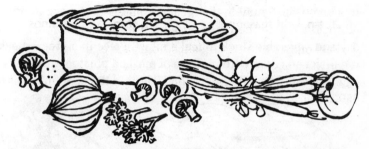

KASHA, GREEN BEAN AND MUSHROOM CASSEROLE

- 1 egg, beaten
- ½ c dark brown buckwheat groats
- 1 tbsp Bragg Aminos
- 1 level tsp Bragg Instant Vegetable Broth Powder
- 1 large onion chopped
- 2 c cooked fresh green beans, sliced
- 1 c grated natural Cheddar cheese
- ½ c celery, finely chopped
- ½ c green pepper, chopped
- 1 can (2-4) oz.) sliced mushrooms, drained
- ¼ c oil
- 1 clove garlic, chopped

Combine egg, groats, Bragg Aminos and Bragg Broth Powder. In medium size frying pan, saute onion, green pepper and mushrooms in oil for four minutes. Stir in groats mixture, green beans and water; bring to a boil.

Cook, tightly covered, over low heat 15 minutes. Turn into serving dish; and then sprinkle cheese over the top.

PEASANT'S PIE

1 egg
½ c whole wheat
   crumbs
1 tsp Italian herbs
1 onion, chopped
2 carrots, grated
1 tbsp soya flour

⅓ c cashew nuts,
   grated
1 tsp sage
   soya oil
½ c vegetable stock
1 tbsp Bragg Liquid
   Aminos

Topping

1 lb mashed potatoes & 1 egg

Chop onions and saute in soya oil till golden. Grate the carrots very fine. Crumble the breadcrumbs, beat the egg and mix all together with the herbs, ground nuts and soya flour. If too dry add vegetable stock to make moist. Place in a greased baking dish and cover with mixture of mashed potatoes and beaten egg. Dot salt-free butter over top if desired. Bake 30 minutes at 350°.

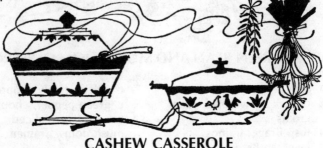

CASHEW CASSEROLE

1 onion, chopped
2 tomatoes, chopped
½ tsp sage
½ c Cheddar Cheese,
   grated
½ tsp Italian herbs

½ c cashew nuts, ground
½ c fresh whole wheat
   breadcrumbs
1 tsp Brewer's Yeast
   soy oil
2 eggs

Peel and chop the onion and cook in soy oil until golden. Skin the tomatoes and chop. Mix together the ground nuts, breadcrumbs, onions, tomatoes, sage, herbs, grated cheese and beaten eggs. Place in a greased baking dish. Bake in 400° oven for 40 to 45 minutes.

BEAN-SQUASH-CASSEROLE

½ lb dry white beans	2 lb spinach or chard
Water	¼ tsp oregano
3 tbsp olive oil	½ c grated Parmesan
3 squash, diced	cheese
3 zucchini, diced	2 tbsp Bragg Aminos
2 cloves garlic,	Yogurt or kefir
sliced	(optional)

Cover beans with water and soak overnight. Add more water if needed and simmer until tender, about 1 hour. Add 1 tablespoon Bragg Aminos just before beans are done. Drain beans and sprinkle with 1 tablespoon of the oil. Heat remaining oil in a deep skillet and add the yellow crookneck and zucchini squashes and garlic. Cook, stirring to prevent scorching, until squashes are tender. Transfer to a greased 3 or 4-quart dish. Wash spinach thoroughly and shake off as much water as possible. If using chard, shred it coarsely. Spread spinach or chard over squash. Top with the beans and season with another tablespoon of Bragg Aminos. Crumble oregano over the top and sprinkle with the cheese. Bake at 350° for 30 to 40 minutes. When about half done stir cheese through vegetable mixture. Serve hot or cold. Top with yogurt or kefir if desired when serving.

FISHLESS "TUNA" CASSEROLE
Linda Barrett's
(With the Unusual Tuna Taste but Fishless)

2 c brown rice, cooked	3 tbsp chopped onion
1 c chopped walnuts	3 tbsp finely chopped
Milk to moisten	celery
½ c whole wheat bread	1 clove garlic, pressed
1 tbsp Bragg Aminos	

Chop onions and celery finely. Mix all the ingredients together thoroughly; add more milk if too dry. Bake in moderate oven (350°) approximately 45 minutes. Then add ½ c lemon juice and let soak in.

EGGPLANT CASSEROLE
Barbara Dendle's

2 medium round eggplant (or 3 or 4 long)
1 large onion, minced
2 large garlic cloves, sliced
1 large can tomato puree (without salt)
Approx. 8 oz thin sliced Monterey Jack cheese
2 tbsp olive oil

Assemble in casserole dish in layers as follows:
Half the eggplant (sliced in ½" slices crosswise)
Half the garlic (sprinkle on top)
Half the tomato puree
Half the onion
Half the cheese
Half the olive oil
Repeat with second layer. Bake in 400° oven for one hour.

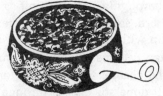

BAKED BEANS
Barbara Dendle's

1 pkg navy beans
8 oz tomato puree
2 tsp dry mustard
1 tsp cinnamon
1 tbsp grated fresh ginger (or 2 tsp. dry)
1 medium onion, chopped
¼ c molasses
1 tsp cloves

Soak beans overnight, having the water about 3 inches above the beans. In the morning boil beans in same water, adding more if necessary. Skim off foam as it comes to the top. Boil until the skins break on the beans. Drain beans, reserving liquid.

Put beans in large casserole with onion. Mix ⅓ of liquid with rest of ingredients and add to beans, saving remainder for adding later.

Bake 300° until done, adding more liquid as beans bake dry.

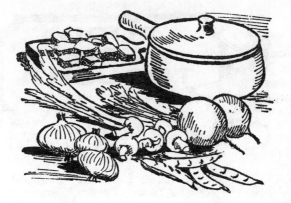

PINTO CASSEROLE

2 c dried pinto beans	¼ c chopped green or
5 c water	sweet red pepper
2 tbsp tomatoes, chopped	1 large clove garlic, minced
& peeled	½ tsp crushed rosemary
2 tsp Bragg Aminos	leaves
1 large onion,	¼ tsp crushed marjoram
coarsely chopped	or oregano

Soak beans overnight in water. Add oil, bring to a boil, reduce heat and simmer, covered, until beans are tender, about 1½ hours. Add tomatoes, onion, green or red pepper, garlic, Bragg Aminos, rosemary and marjoram or oregano. Turn into a greased baking dish and bake at 325° for 1 hour.

UNCOMPLICATE YOUR LIVING

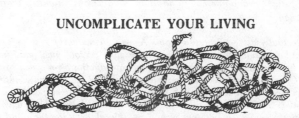

Living is a continual lesson in problem solving, but the trick is to know where to start. No excuses — start your Health Program Today.

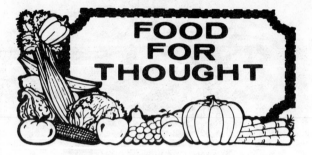

FOOD FOR THOUGHT

Thomson, in his poem, "The Seasons," written two hundred and twenty-four years ago, pays the following tribute to a diet composed of seeds and vegetable products: —

"With such a liberal hand has Nature flung
 These seeds abroad, blown them about in winds —
 But who their virtues can declare? who pierce,
 With vision pure, into those secret stores
 Of health and life and joy — the food of man,
 While yet he lived in innocence and told
 A length of golden years, unfleshed in blood?
 A stranger to the savage arts of life —
 Death, rapine, carnage, surfeit, and disease —
 The lord, and not the tyrant of the world."

Most assuredly I do believe that body and mind are much influenced by the kind of food habitually depended upon. I can never stray among the village people of our windy capes without now and then coming upon a human being who looks as if he had been split, salted, and dried, like the salt fish which has built up his arid organism. If the body is modified by the food which nourishes it, the mind and character very certainly will be modified by it also. We know enough of their close connection with each other to be sure of that without any statistical observation to prove it.
                                                              — Oliver Wendell Holmes

The word "vegetarian" is not derived from "vegetable," but from the Latin, homo vegetus, meaning among the Romans a strong, robust, thoroughly healthy man.

An intellectual feast — Professor Louis Agassiz in his early manhood visited Germany to consult Oken, the transcendentalist in zoological classification. "After I had delivered to him my letter of introduction," he once said to a friend, "Oken asked me to dine with him, and you may suppose with what joy I accepted the invitation. The dinner consisted only of potatoes, boiled and roasted; but it was the best dinner I ever ate; for there was Oken. Never before were such potatoes grown on this planet; for the mind of the man seemed to enter into what we ate sociably together, and I devoured his intellect while munching his potatoes."

110

ENTREES

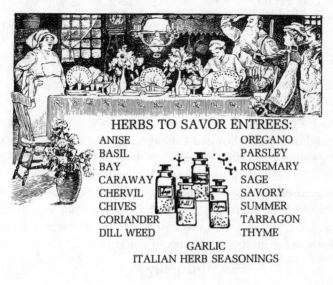

HERBS TO SAVOR ENTREES:

ANISE	OREGANO
BASIL	PARSLEY
BAY	ROSEMARY
CARAWAY	SAGE
CHERVIL	SAVORY
CHIVES	SUMMER
CORIANDER	TARRAGON
DILL WEED	THYME

GARLIC
ITALIAN HERB SEASONINGS

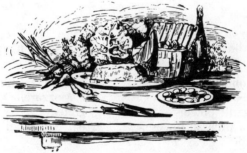

DANISH WALNUT AND CHEESE LOAF
Ellen Andreasen's

½	green pepper, chopped	1½ c bread crumbs
½	large onion, chopped	½ c tomato sauce
2½ c	grated cheese	6 eggs
⅓ c	milk	1 tbsp Bragg Aminos
2 c	chopped walnuts	

Mix ingredients and press lightly into a 2-quart casserole.
Bake at 325° for 1 hour.

HAZELNUT PIE

½ c Hazelnuts, ground
1½ c Cheddar Cheese,
   grated
1 tsp Italian herbs

1 tbsp Bragg Aminos
2 eggs
½ c Shreddies or crushed
   Shredded Wheat

Filling

2 large onions
   soy oil

½ medium cabbage

Peel, chop and saute the onions in the soy oil, adding the washed and well chopped cabbage, and cook till tender. Mix the ground hazelnuts, cheese, crushed Shreddies and beaten eggs with the Italian herbs and Aminos. Place half the mixture in a greased baking dish. On top of this place the onion and cabbage mixture and top this with the remaining nut mixture. Pack down and dot with raw salt-free butter if desired. Bake in 400° oven for 30 to 45 minutes or till golden.

RICE PIZZA

Crust

3 c brown rice, cooked
2 eggs, beaten

Topping

16 oz Tomato sauce,
   Fresh or canned
⅓ tsp garlic powder
2 tbsp Parmesan Cheese,
   grated

1 c Mozzarella Cheese,
   grated
1 tsp Bragg Aminos
1 c Mozzarella Cheese,
   grated
½ tsp Italian herbs

To make crust, combine rice, eggs, and cheese. Press firmly into a 12-inch greased pizza pan (or two, 9-inch pie pans) by spreading evenly with a spatula. Bake at 450° for 20 minutes. For the topping combine tomato sauce and seasonings. Spread evenly over rice crust. Top with Mozzarella and Parmesan cheeses. Bake 10 minutes longer. To serve, cut in wedges. You may use the following as additional topping, if desired: finely sliced onion rings, mushrooms, red or green bell peppers, and sliced black olives. This as the entree with a big health salad first—makes a delicious meal.

RICE, CAULIFLOWER AND POTATO MIX

1½ c long-grain brown rice	3¾ c hot water
1 medium-size potato	1¼ tsp hot water
	1 tsp Bragg Aminos
⅔ small cauliflower	¼ tsp allspice powder
2 tbsp soy oil	⅛ tsp ginger powder
¼ tsp caraway seeds	¼ tsp parsley flakes
	¼ tsp mustard seeds

Wash rice thoroughly 3 times in separate container. Wash and cut potato (skin is best part) into small pieces, break cauliflower into flowerets and add to rice. Place grease in large saucepan and add caraway seeds and mustard seeds. Fry 1 minute, until spices are lightly browned, then quickly add rice, cauliflower and potato. Saute 1 minute, stirring constantly. Add hot water, stir again and add Bragg Aminos and remaining spices. Cook on medium heat 10-12 minutes or until water stops bubbling up through rice. Turn off heat, cover pot completely and let stand 5-7 minutes.

GOURMET MEAT BALLS

1 c Walnuts	1 can tomato paste, or fresh
2 cloves garlic	
1 onion	1 can tomato sauce, or fresh
1 carrot	
1 tbsp celery	1 tbsp apple cider vinegar
2 tbsp parsley	
2 tsp Bragg Aminos	1 c water
⅓ c whole wheat bread crumbs	2 tbsp onions, minced
	2 tbsp green pepper, minced
2 eggs	
3 tbsp soy oil	1 bay leaf

Grind walnuts, garlic, onion, celery, carrot and parsley together. Add 1 tsp Bragg Aminos, ⅓ cup dry bread crumbs and eggs. Then shape into balls. Saute balls until browned on all sides in soy oil. Combine tomato sauce, paste, apply cider vinegar, water, onions, green pepper and bay leaf. Add meat balls and simmer 1 hour. Serve over brown rice.

MIXED NUTS AND BEANS

½ c mixed raw nuts, chopped
½ c soya beans, cooked
1 Spanish onion, large
2 tbsp soy oil

½ c Lima beans, cooked
½ c String beans, cooked
½ c Yogurt
1 tsp Honey

Peel and slice the onion and saute in Soy Oil until golden. Add the beans and nuts, stir in the yogurt, and honey. Serve either as it is or on plain steamed brown rice.

CURRY RICE
Ingrid Klingler's

3 c brown rice (soak all day or overnight)
½ tsp curry powder

1 tbsp olive oil
5 cloves garlic, pressed
3¾ c water

Bring above ingredients to a boil, then turn down heat, simmer for 20-25 min. Serve with lemon or Bragg Aminos.

SYRIAN THETCHOUKA

6 eggs
3 spanish onions, sliced
3 cloves garlic, minced
½ c Cheddar Cheese, grated
1 tbsp Bragg Aminos
3 green or red bell peppers, chop seeds also

4 tbsp olive oil
3 tomatoes, chopped
1 carrot, coarse grated
2 tbsp Parmesan Cheese, grated

Peel and slice the onions and saute them in the olive oil until golden. Add the garlic and the other vegetables sliced and the Bragg Aminos. Put the lid on the pan and cook gently until all the vegetables are tender. Transfer the mixture to a greased casserole with lid, make 6 hollows in the mixture and carefully drop an egg into each one. Sprinkle with the grated cheese and bake for 10 minutes or until the eggs are set.

114

ECONOMY "NO MEAT" HAMBURGERS

2 eggs, beaten
½ c walnuts, ground
1 c oatmeal, uncooked
3 tbsp water
½ c onions, minced

½ tsp sage
1 tsp Bragg Aminos
1 clove garlic, pressed
2 tbsp soy oil
½ c water

Combine eggs, walnuts, uncooked oatmeal, 3 tbsp water, onion, sage, garlic and Bragg Aminos. Stir and blend well then form into patties. Brown patties on both sides in soy oil. Add water then cover skillet and simmer until the liquid is almost evaporated.

RICE-STUFFED CABBAGE

1 Head cabbage, medium
1 c water
2 tbsp Soy Oil
5 Green Onions,
   thinly sliced
½ c brown rice
½ c parsley, minced

1 tbsp Bragg Aminos
½ tsp cinnamon
½ c chopped walnuts
4 whole cloves
6 carrots
2 Tomatoes, peeled
   & diced

Place cabbage in deep pot of rapidly boiling water, cover and blanch for 5 minutes. Remove cabbage from water, drain well and carefully spread leaves as if opening flower petals. Cut a large piece from center. Heat Soy Oil in skillet, add green onions and cook until tender. Add rice and cook until it appears translucent. Add parsley, tomatoes, water, aminos and cinnamon. Cover tightly and cook 25 minutes. Most of the liquid should be absorbed but rice will not be tender at this point. Chop center portion of cabbage and add to rice along with walnuts. Carefully spoon stuffing into center of cabbage and between leaves. Shape into head again and tie securely with clean string. Place in deep pot. Stud cabbage with whole cloves. Cut carrots into two or three pieces each and place around cabbage. Add 1 cup boiling water. Cover and simmer on top of range or in oven at 325° until tender. Cut into wedges to serve.

TRINIDAD MOCK DUCK

½ lb soya beans, cooked
½ lb lentils, cooked
1 small onion, chopped
1 c cooked potatoes
   Sweet basil leaves

3 tbsp butter, salt-free
2 tbsp parsley, chopped
½ tsp fresh or dry sage
1 tbsp Bragg Aminos
   Tomato Juice as required

Add the cooked soya beans to the lentils and the mashed potatoes. Saute the onion in half the raw butter and add the soya bean mixture. Add sage, sweet basil, chopped parsley and season with Bragg Aminos. Shape into size of small tennis balls, put on a greased baking dish, pour over balance of (melted) butter, and bake in 350° oven until deep brown. Serve in a hot tureen with lots of hot, thickened tomato juice. (Pre-thicken with whole wheat flour)

LENTILS WITH WALNUTS

2 c lentils
2 tbsp butter, salt-free

¾ c ground walnuts
¼ tsp Italian herb
   seasonings

Cook lentils until tender and quite dry. Put through colander or mash. Add ground walnuts and herbs. Put in greased casserole and bake 20 to 30 minutes. Serves 3.

LENTILS WITH WILD RICE
OR WHOLE-GRAIN CEREAL

1¼ c lentils, puréed
2 tbsp butter, salt-free
½ c milk or soy milk
2 eggs
1 small onion, minced

1½ c cooked wild rice
   or whole-grain cereal
¼ c chives
½ tsp rosemary

Combine lentils and wild rice (or whole-grain cereal); add butter, milk. Separate yolks and whites of eggs. Beat whites until stiff. Stir yolks into mixture and fold in whites with herbs. Place in buttered casserole in moderate oven, watching carefully until mixture is well set and top delicately brown. Serves 4.

116

LIMA-BEAN LOAF

1 egg, slightly beaten
1½ tbsp butter or soy
   or olive oil
1 c dried lima beans
1 lemon, juice only

1½ c whole-wheat cracker
   crumbs
1 tbsp minced pimiento
1 c milk or soy milk

Wash and soak the beans overnight. Cook until soft, drain, and rub through a coarse sieve. Mix the other ingredients, place in greased casserole, and bake in a moderate oven. Baste with lemon juice and butter. Serves 5. May be prepared also with cooked whole-grain cereals instead of lima beans.

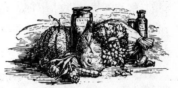

SOYBEAN LOAF

3 c soybeans
3 eggs
3 tbsp grated onion
¾ c water

¾ c whole-wheat crackers
¾ c milk or soy milk
6 tbsp butter or oil
1½ tbsp grated orange
   or lemon peel

Cook and mash the beans. Brown the whole-wheat cracker crumbs and sift. Mix all ingredients together thoroughly. Place in a greased bread pan and bake 30 minutes in a moderate oven. Serve hot or cold. Serves 8.

VEGETARIAN LOAF

1½ c cooked peas
1½ c cooked beans
1½ c cooked brown rice
   or whole-grain cereal

3 tbsp melted butter
2¼ c tomato sauce
⅛ tsp celery seed
3 eggs, beaten

Use fresh or dry beans and peas. While hot put them through a food-chopper. Add all the other ingredients but the hot sauce and shape into a loaf, adding more cooked brown rice or cereal if necessary. Season to taste. Bake in a moderate oven for 45 minutes. Serve with hot tomato sauce. Serves 8.

BEAN PATTIES

1 c whole-wheat bread crumbs
1 beaten egg

2 c cooked or canned beans
1 tbsp chopped parsley

Mix the above ingredients and form into patties. Bake for about 10 minutes. Any legumes may be used in this recipe. Serves 4.

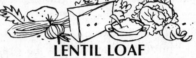

LENTIL LOAF

1½ c whole-wheat bread crumbs
1 c milk or soy milk
2 tbsp olive, or soy oil

1½ tbsp chopped parsley
¾ tsp sage
1½ c cooked lentils
2 garlic cloves, mashed

Mix the above ingredients well, put into greased pan, and bake in a moderate oven until firm. Beans or peas may be substituted for lentils. Cooked whole-grain cereal may be used in place of lentils. Serves 5.

LENTIL RISSOLES

2 c lentils, cooked
2 onions, chopped
1 egg
½ c whole wheat bread crumbs
½ c fresh whole wheat breadcrumbs, browned

soy oil
2 oz Cheddar Cheese, grated
1 tsp Italian herbs
1 tsp Bragg Liquid Aminos

Peel, chop and saute the onions in Soy Oil till tender and golden. Boil the lentils in sufficient boiling water till tender. Drain well any excess moisture. Mix all ingredients together and cool. Form the cold mixture into rissoles and roll well in the breadcrumbs. Bake in 425° oven on a well-heated baking tray just covered with Soy Oil. Turn over the rissoles at 15 minutes and cook for further 15 minutes.

The unexamined life is not worth living. It is time to re-evaluate your past as a guide to your future. —Socrates

BAKED VEGETABLE LOAF

1 egg	1 c chopped, stewed prunes
1 c milk	1 c peas
dash of fresh ground	¼ c unsulphured molasses
peppercorn	2 c diced carrots
½ green pepper	1 c diced potatoes
½ onion	1 c whole-wheat bread
2 tbsp melted butter	crumbs

Cook carrots and potatoes, chop coarse, and mix with chopped green pepper and chopped onion; add peas and prunes. Add all the seasonings, beaten egg, butter, and molasses. Mix thoroughly, place in buttered baking pan, and bake in a hot oven about 400° for 1 hour. Serves 6.

VEGETARIAN SAUSAGES

2 c cooked soybeans	⅛ tsp powdered sage
1 c cooked lima beans	1 egg
1 c cooked navy beans	1 c cornmeal or whole-
⅛ tsp paprika	wheat cracker crumbs
⅔ c milk or soy milk	1 tsp poultry seasoning
1 tbsp Bragg Liquid Aminos	1 tbsp butter, salt-free

Press the beans through a colander and mix in all the seasonings. Beat the egg with milk. Shape seasoned beans into sausage shapes, and bake in 400° oven until top is browned, about 20 minutes. Serves 8.

BASIC KIDNEY BEANS

1 c dried red kidney beans	2 cloves garlic (optional)
1 tsp Bragg Aminos	1 tsp Bragg Instant
1 large onion, chopped	Vegetable Broth Powder
1 tbsp olive oil	1 bayleaf

Combine ingredients in stewing pan and bring to boil. Cook over medium heat 1½ hours.

Rev. Fawn Jacquelin Higgs (Haleiwa, Hawaii 96712) is noted for her unusual and creative recipes. She is a master at the vegetarian cuisine and is the author of a new outstanding cookbook titled OUR DAILY BREAD. Following are three of her delicious and nutritious recipes:

MUSHROOM BURGERS
Rev. Fawn Higgs

1 c cooked garbanzos, drained	1 large egg
½ c onion finely chopped	¾ c wheat germ
1½ c chopped mushrooms (fresh)	2 tsp Bragg Aminos

Mash garbanzos in medium size bowl with fork, add ¼ c of wheat germ and rest of ingredients and mix by hand thoroughly. Form into burgers and roll in rest of wheat germ. Saute in just enough vegetable oil or butter to cover the bottom of the pan. Brown slowly on both sides over medium heat.

BROWN RICE CHINESE STYLE
Rev. Fawn Higgs

2 c brown rice, cooked	½ c chopped onion
1 c chopped bean sprouts	2 hard-boiled eggs, chopped
½ c chopped water chestnuts (fresh or canned)	1 tsp anise seed
3 tbsp unsalted butter or or vegetable oil	2 tbsp Bragg Aminos with 2 tbsp water
½ c chopped stringed celery	

Heat butter in skillet. Add rice, then rest of ingredients. Mix well over medium hot pan. Entire operation should not take more than 5 to 8 min. Mushrooms may be added if desired.

If a man can convince me that I do not think or act right, gladly will I change, for I search after truth. But he is harmed who abideth on still in his ignorance.
—Marcus Aurelius, Roman Emporer

NUT BURGERS
Rev. Fawn Higgs

1 c chopped pecans
½ c macadamia nut bits (or finely chopped almonds)
½ c chopped pine nuts
2 eggs
⅔ c chopped stringed celery
1 c cooked white cornmeal (stiff)

⅔ c wheat germ
3 tsp poultry seasoning
2 tsp thyme
2 tbsp Bragg Aminos
½ stick melted butter
⅔ c black walnuts coarse chopped

Mix cornmeal, wheat germ, eggs and Bragg Aminos well. Add rest of ingredients in bowl suitable for mixing. Pour butter on top and mix thoroughly by hand. Beat eggs first (no need to separate the whites) to ensure thorough mixing. Form into round burgers, roll in wheat germ and saute in vegetable oil (should be pre-heated). When suitably browned, remove from pan and put on paper towelling to absorb extra grease. Can be served hot or cold.

STUFFED PEPPERS ROYAL
Pete and Marj's

2 c cooked soybeans
2 tbsp chopped onion
1 tbsp melted butter
1 c chopped pepper
1 tbsp Bragg Instant Vegetable Broth Powder
1 c finely chopped walnut meats
1 c grated Cheddar Cheese

½ c tomato juice
½ tsp sage
1 c chopped celery
1 tbsp Bragg Aminos

Prepare peppers by removing seeds and covering with boiling water. Bring to rapid boil and drain. Mash soybeans and add other ingredients. Fill pepper shells with soybean stuffing and add ½ tsp. of paprika to each. Place stuffed peppers in casserole in which ½ inch water from the peppers is included.

Cover and bake for 45 minutes at 400°. During the last 5 minutes, uncover and generously sprinkle grated Cheddar Cheese over each pepper.

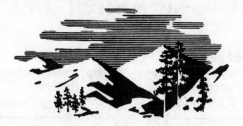

TEN HEALTH COMMANDMENTS

Thou shall respect thy body as the highest manifestation of Life.

Thou shall abstain from all unnatural, devitalized food and stimulating beverages.

Thou shall nourish thy body with only Natural, unprocessed, "live" food, —that

Thou shall extend thy years in health for loving, charitable service.

Thou shall regenerate thy body by the right balance of activity and rest.

Thou shall purify thy cells, tissue and blood with pure fresh air and sunshine.

Thou shall abstain from ALL food when out of sorts in mind or body.

Thou shall keep thy thoughts, words and emotions, pure, calm and uplifting.

Thou shall increase thy knowledge of Nature's laws, abide therewith, and enjoy the fruits of thy life's labor.

Thou shall lift up thyself and thy brother with thine own obedience to ALL Nature's laws.

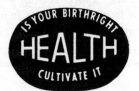

122

EGG & CHEESE DISHES

HERBS TO SAVOR EGGS–CHEESES:

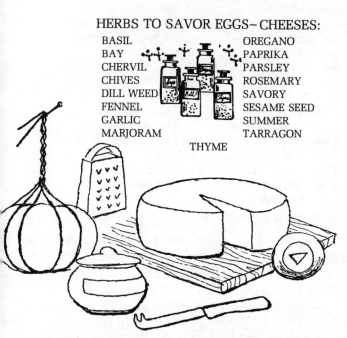

BASIL	OREGANO
BAY	PAPRIKA
CHERVIL	PARSLEY
CHIVES	ROSEMARY
DILL WEED	SAVORY
FENNEL	SESAME SEED
GARLIC	SUMMER
MARJORAM	TARRAGON

THYME

VEGETARIAN MOCK CHOPPED CHICKEN LIVER
Fred and Jean Pump's

1 tbsp Bragg Aminos   1 clove pressed garlic
½ c finely chopped onion   3 tbsp olive oil
1 pound cooked green beans, chopped extremely fine
3 hard-boiled eggs, finely mashed
1 c finely chopped mushrooms

Saute onions, mushrooms, and garlic in olive oil. When done, add the finely chopped cooked string beans and the finely chopped hard-boiled eggs.

Mix thoroughly with the hands. Chill 1 hour before serving.

HEALTH in a human being, is the perfection of bodily organization, intellectual energy, and moral power.

GHIVETCH WITH CHEESE

1 c carrots,
thinly sliced

1 c snap beans,
diagonally cut

½ c celery, thinly
sliced

2 tomatoes, peeled
& quartered

1 Yellow Summer Squash,
thinly sliced

1 Zucchini, thinly
sliced

½ onion, thinly sliced

⅓ bay leaf, crumbled

½ head cauliflower,
broken in flowerets

½ sweet red pepper,
cut in strips

½ c shelled green peas

⅓ c Olive or Soy Oil

3 cloves garlic, minced

2 tsp Bragg Aminos

½ tsp savory crushed

½ tsp tarragon, crushed

Grated Parmesan
Cheese

Jack or Swiss Cheese,
cut in strips

Combine all vegetables in a shallow baking dish. Heat broth & add oil, garlic, Aminos, bay leaf, savory and tarragon. Bring broth mixture to a boil, pour over vegetables and cover casserole tightly. Bake at 350° for 1 hour or until vegetables are tender. Gently stir vegetables twice while cooking. Uncover casserole, sprinkle generously with Parmesan Cheese and cover with strips of Jack or Swiss Cheese. Broil until bubbly.

BAKED EGGPLANT FRITATTA

2 Large Eggplants

4 eggs

1 tsp Bragg Aminos

½ c water or
milk
soy oil

1 c Parmesan and Romano Cheese mixed, grated

½ c wheat germ or fine dry whole wheat crumbs

Prick unpeeled eggplants at intervals with a fork. Broil, turning often, until skin is shriveled (or bake eggplants at 450° until skin is shriveled). Cool eggplant, strip off skin and chop or mash the pulp fine. Mix with ¾ cup of the cheese, wheat germ or crumbs, eggs, water or milk, and Bragg Aminos. (You may chop up skin and add to mixture—it's optional.) Turn into a well-greased baking dish. Sprinkle with remaining cheese and a little oil. Bake at 350° for 25 minutes or until a knife inserted in center comes out clean.

EGGPLANT STUFFED WITH EGG

1 Large Eggplant	1 tsp Bragg Aminos
2 tbsp Soy Oil	1 tbsp Lemon Juice
1 onion, minced	3 hard-boiled eggs,
1 green pepper,	chopped fine
chopped	Wheat Germ
2 tomatoes, peeled	½ tsp Kelp Seasoning
and chopped	1 clove garlic, minced

Wash and dry eggplant, cut in halves lengthwise and scoop out pulp, leaving half shells ½ in. thick. Cover with water and let stand while preparing stuffing. Heat oil in large skillet. Add onion, green pepper and garlic and cook until tender but not browned. Add tomatoes and eggplant pulp, which has been chopped fine. Cook until tender, mashing in pan to form a paste. Stir in Bragg Liquid Aminos, kelp seasoning, lemon juice and eggs. Drain eggplant shells and fill with mixture. Sprinkle with wheat germ. Place in a shallow baking dish. Bake in 350° oven for 25 minutes.

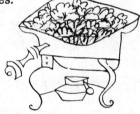

BROCCOLI MAIN DISH

1½ lbs broccoli	1 tbsp Bragg Aminos
2 eggs	2 tbsp soy oil
1 c cottage cheese	⅓ c whole wheat
¼ c green onion,	bread crumbs
minced	2 tbsp Parmesan cheese,
¼ c Cheddar Cheese	grated

Trim stems of broccoli, then blanch in boiling water for 5 minutes. Drain broccoli then lay in well-oiled baking dish. Combined the eggs, cottage cheese, green onion, cheeses and Bragg Aminos. Pour this mixture over broccoli. Combine 2 tablespoons of soy oil and whole wheat bread crumbs and sprinkle on top of casserole. Bake in 350° oven for 25 minutes.

CHEESE ALMOND CASSEROLE

1 c mushrooms, sliced,
   fresh
2 tsp minced onions
2 tsp green peppers,
   minced
⅓ c almonds, chopped

2 tbsp Soy Oil
1¼ c brown rice
2 tbsp Bragg Aminos
3½ c water
¾ c Cheddar Cheese,
   grated

Place Soy Oil in skillet and saute mushrooms, onions and green peppers until slightly tender. Then add almonds, brown rice, and aminos. Combine these ingredients then turn into a casserole. Pour 3½ cups water into casserole. Stir. Then top with grated Cheddar Cheese and bake, covered in a 350° oven for 45 minutes.

CHEDDAR CHEESE AND LENTIL BAKE

2 c Lentils, cooked
6 oz Cheddar Cheese,
   grated
1 tsp Brewer's Yeast
1 tbsp Bragg Liquid Aminos

2 onions, chopped
2 eggs
Soy Oil
2 fresh tomatoes
   (optional)

Peel, chop and saute the onions in Soy Oil till golden. Cook the lentils in sufficient boiling water till tender; drain any excess moisture. Mix the lentils with the onions, grated cheese, beaten eggs, Aminos and Brewer's Yeast. Put in a greased baking dish. Arrange on top the skinned and thinly sliced tomatoes. Bake in 400° oven for 30 to 45 minutes.

SPROUTED SOYBEAN OMELET

4 eggs
4 tbsp milk (soy or cow's)
½ c green onion tops

2 tbsp butter, salt free
2 c sprouted soybeans

Beat whole eggs lightly, adding milk and seasoning. Melt the butter in the omelet pan. Pour in mixture, bean sprouts and chopped onion tops. Lift cooked part slightly from time to time, to allow the uncooked part to run under it and brown. Allow pan to heat quickly so that it will brown quickly. Serves 6.

HARDBOILED EGGS, OLIVE OIL AND PRESSED GARLIC

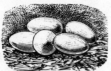

This is a quick and convenient way to extract the high protein found in eggs, particularly fertile eggs, if you can obtain them.

Hard boil two or more eggs. Cool. Remove shells. Mash eggs with a fork and add 2 tbsp olive oil and 1 or 2 cloves of pressed garlic. Mix eggs, oil and garlic thoroughly. (Note: This can be eaten with celery sticks, sliced cabbage, 100% whole wheat toast, whole wheat wafers or Norwegian crisp rye squares. I find dark Ry-King very tasty.) A medium salad with this followed by fresh fruit for dessert, makes a balanced nutritional meal.

MASHED AVOCADO, OLIVE OIL AND PRESSED GARLIC

1 medium sized avocado	1 small clove garlic,
1 tbsp olive oil	pressed

Mash avocado with a fork and add the oil and garlic, mixing thoroughly.

Use same combinations as given in the previous recipe, HARD BOILED EGGS, OLIVE OIL AND PRESSED GARLIC.

CHEESE NUT LOAF

1 c brown rice, cooked	1 lb Cheddar Cheese, grated
1 c wheat germ	1 clove garlic, minced
1½ c walnuts, chopped	1 tsp Bragg Aminos
1 onion, minced	½ c mushrooms,
4 eggs, beaten	thinly sliced

Combine rice, wheat germ, walnuts, onion, mushrooms, cheese, garlic, Bragg Aminos in a large bowl. Mix well, add eggs and mix thoroughly. Pack mixture into a well-greased loaf pan. Bake in 350° oven for 50 minutes or until firm. Remove from oven and let stand 10 minutes then carefully loosen at sides with knife and turn out onto a warm platter. Slice and serve.

CHEESE POLENTA

1 c yellow cornmeal, stone ground	3 tbsp soy oil
3½ c boiling water	1 egg, beaten
2 tbsp onion, minced	½ c Parmesan cheese, grated
1 tsp Bragg Aminos	½ c Cheddar cheese, grated

Add cornmeal to boiling water very, very slowly. Stir constantly. Then stir in onion, Bragg Aminos, soy oil, egg and ½ cup of mixed cheeses. Pour into 9" x 9" baking dish. Sprinkle remaining cheese over top and put under broiler 4 minutes.

CHEESE CAKE
Barbara Dendle's

Blend thoroughly together:

6 eggs	4 tsp unsalted butter
2 tbsp lemon juice	½ cup honey (generous)
2 tsp pure vanilla	

Add: 32 ounces (large carton) cottage cheese

Blend until very smooth. Pour into pan (loaf style or square). Top with cinnamon. Bake in pre-heated 350° oven until firm.

Turn off oven, leave cake there with door open for one hour more, then chill.

This may be served plain or topped with berries, fruit or applesauce.

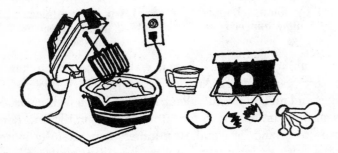

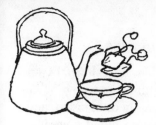

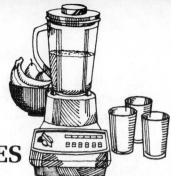

HEALTH BEVERAGES

All over the United States we hear about the "cocktail hours" for which beautifully colored creations of liquor are invented to produce new thrills, to stimulate jaded appetites and bolster up failing spirits.

Now we have a new kind of "cocktail." It is not made of whisky or gin. There isn't a pickled cherry to be found in one of them. They are made from fresh young vegetables and ripe fruits — the very blood of the plant. There is no liquor on the face of the earth so satisfying as the tomato, grapefruit or orange juice cocktail. Not only is it delicious but a cocktail made of fresh vegetable and fruit juice is a brilliantly colorful sight as it sparkles in a crystal cocktail glass. And there is something more — more than satisfying the palate and the eye — the satisfaction and nourishment of the billions of the cells of which the body is composed. When people take to the Health cocktail habit, they put liquid life into their bodies.

When we consider that fruits and vegetables have been naturally cooked by solar energy, they they contain all of the elements that the sun and the earth have buried deep into their fibrous cells, that they are live cell food, is it not reasonable that if we crush the precious juices from the cells of these fresh fruits and vegetables, we will receive vital energy from them?

HOW TO SELECT AND PREPARE FOOD FOR JUICING

In selecting foods with which to make the best Health cocktails, choose the deep-colored, young, tender, heavier, more solid fruits and fresh vegetables. They contain more juice. Use both the leaves and stems as well as the body of the vegetables. They yield an abundance of organic minerals. The tops of the carrots, for instance, contain phosphorus.

129

FRUIT AND VEGETABLE DRINKS

Fruit and vegetable juices can be purchased fresh from your Health food store or prepared at home with some type of juice extractor. The juices can be used individually or blended, and with a dash of herbs, particularly in tomato blend combinations, make an inspiring Health drink. Here are some excellent combinations:

(NOTE: In using herbs in these drinks, use only 1 or 2 crushed leaves if fresh, and a very small pinch if the herbs are dried.)

1. Tomato, celery, and basil
2. Tomato, celery, and chives
3. Tomato, celery, cucumber, basil and garlic
4. Tomato, spinach, and mint
5. Tomato, celery, and watercress
6. Grapefruit and orange
7. Beet, parsley, and cucumber
8. Beet, celery, and carrot
9. Cucumber and pineapple
10. Carrot, tomato, and mint
11. Cucumber, watercress, and carrot
12. Carrot, celery, and marjoram
13. Carrot and coconut milk
14. Carrot, celery and spinach
15. Carrot and rosemary
16. Carrot, parsley and tomato
17. Apple, pineapple and mint
18. Plum and apple
19. Papaya and plum
20. Papaya and nectarine
21. Papaya and grape juice

OTHER HEALTHFUL DRINKS

HERB TEA

Many delicious herb teas can be brewed, among them the very popular mint tea. Simply take mint leaves and brew as you would any ordinary tea.

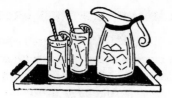

SPICED MINT TEA

3⅓ c water
1 3-inch stick cinnamon
6 whole allspice
6 whole cloves
2⅔ tbsp mint tea leaves

⅔ c honey
⅔ c orange juice, fresh
⅓ c lemon juice, fresh
⅓ c grape juice

Combine water and spices in saucepan; bring to bubbling boil. Pour water and spices over tea leaves; steep 5 minutes, strain. Add honey, stirring until well mixed. Cover and cool. Add fresh juices last and serve in freezer chilled glasses. Serves 2 to 3.

PINEAPPLE MINT JULEP

4 sprigs fresh mint
½ c honey
½ c lemon juice, fresh

2¼ c pineapple juice, unsweetened

Wash mint leaves, bruise with spoon; cover with honey. Add lemon juice and let stand about 15 minutes. Add pineapple juice and mix. Pour over ice in pitcher or tall glasses. Garnish with sprigs of mint. Makes about 6 glasses.

MINT DELIGHT

¾ c water
¾ c honey
¾ c lime juice, fresh

2¼ c grapefruit juice, fresh
18 sprigs mint, chopped

Combine water, honey; simmer 8 minutes. Pour over the chopped mint leaves. Cool; stir into combined fruit juices. Pour over ice in tall glasses. Serve right away.

131

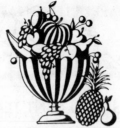

APRICOT AMBROSIA PUNCH

⅓ lb dried unsulphured
   apricots
⅔ c apple juice,
   unsweetened

⅔ c lemon juice, fresh
½ c honey
⅔ c fresh orange juice

Cook apricots until tender; then press fruit and juice through sieve. Add honey and fruit juices and mix well. Chill. Just before serving, pour over ice in punch bowl. Garnish with orange and lemon slices. Makes 16 punch-cup servings.

HONEY PUNCH

½ c honey
2 c water
2 c grape juice,
   unsweetened
¼ c lemon juice, fresh

¼ c cherry juice
1 c pineapple juice
1 mashed banana
½ c apricot pulp

Blend thoroughly, adding a few ice cubes to mixture to chill, and serve. Serves 3.

BARLEY WATER

Wash ¼ cup natural barley and let soak overnight.
Add 1 quart of water and boil gently until the barley is thoroughly done and the liquid is reduced to about 1½ cups. Strain and serve plain or add milk. Season to taste.

Some students drink deeply at the fountain of knowledge—others only gargle.

APPLE LEMONADE

6 c apple juice,   fresh mint sprigs
   unsweetened   1⅛ c lemon juice, unstrained
½ c honey

Combine apple juice and lemon juice. Add honey and stir until it dissolves. Fill 5 or 6 glasses about ⅔ full with the apple lemonade; then add enough ice to fill the glasses. Place a sprig of fresh mint leaves in each glass. Serves 8.

GRAPEFRUIT FOAM

Beat an egg white until stiff. Add 2 teaspoons honey and beat thoroughly. Add 3 cups grapefruit juice and pour into glasses. Sprinkle with a dash of cinnamon or nutmeg. Makes 4 servings.

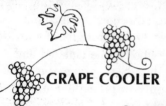

GRAPE COOLER

1 c honey   2 c orange juice, fresh
3 c water   1 c lemon juice, fresh
2 c grape juice

Make a syrup of the honey and water; let cool. Add fruit juices. Pour over ice in pitcher or tall glasses. Serves 12.

Simplicity . . . simplicity . . . simplicity, let your affairs be as two or three, and not as a hundred or a thousand.

Perfect health is above gold, and a sound body before riches. *Solomon*

The laws of health are inexorable; we see people going down and out in the prime of life simply because no attention is paid to them.   *– Bragg*

PINEAPPLE HOLDS THE SECRET OF PROTEIN-DIGESTING ENZYMES

As a nutritionist with over 60 years of practice, I have found that many people do not get the benefit of the protein they eat, whether animal or vegetable proteins.

When I first came to the Hawaiian Islands in 1912, I discovered that the native Hawaiians were digesting their proteins perfectly. And so I studied their eating habits very carefully and learned that the Hawaiians ate fresh pineapple with almost every meal. In further research, I found that the pineapple contained a powerful protein-digesting enzyme.

One of the greatest breakthroughs of nutrition is that this protein-digesting enzyme can be isolated and used as a digestant. This digestant has been given the name "bromelain." Bromelain is found only in pineapple and therefore everyone should make it a point to eat pineapple as often as he can get it fresh. Besides the delectable taste and vitamin and mineral content (vitamins A, E, C and the B complex, and calcium, phosphorus, iron, copper and magnesium), pineapples contain powerful protein digesting enzymes.

I find that if the meal is begun with a slice of fresh pineapple or about 4 oz. of unsweetened pineapple juice, the bromelain in the pineapple will speedily help to digest the proteins wherever they are found—in eggs, fish, meat, cheese, beans, nuts or seeds.

In nutritional laboratories, bromelain has been extracted from fresh pineapple, made into a powder and placed in capsules. These capsules are available at health food stores and may be taken after meals to aid in the digestion of protein.

Here in Hawaii many tasty protein drinks are made from pineapple called "smoothies." Here are the Bragg favorites:

PINEAPPLE AMBROSIA PROTEIN SMOOTHIE

1 tsp Brewer's yeast   1 banana
1 yolk of an egg   1 tbsp honey
1 tsp raw wheat germ
6 oz. unsweetened pineapple juice (freshly squeezed when
    possible) or 1 c fresh pineapple chopped

Blend all of the ingredients in a blender and you have a
perfect protein drink. You may blend in an ice cube to cool and
pour into freezer frosted glasses.

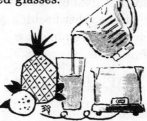

In Hawaii six mornings a week I conduct the Longer Life,
Health and Happiness Club on the grassy compound of Fort
DeRussy at Waikiki Beach. This group of health minded people
jog, do the Bragg super-brain breathing, the orthopedic exer-
cises, and finish their workout with a swim.

Bill Stenjem, one of my associate instructors, has developed
an excellent blender protein drink as follows:

HI-PROTEIN SMOOTHIE
Bill Stenjem's

1 tbsp low fat soy powder   1 tbsp Brewer's yeast
1 tbsp flaxseed meal   powder
1 tbsp rice polishings   2 tbsp raw honey
⅓ pt plain yogurt   1-2 ripe bananas
    handful of alfalfa sprouts
2 c unsweetened pineapple juice or fresh pineapple

(Note: All of these ingredients can be purchased at your health
        food store.)
Bill is a powerhouse of health and energy and shows by precept
and example that the natural health life pays off handsomely.
Here are two more delicious pineapple protein drinks:

135

CAROB SMOOTHIE
(Chocolate flavor)

1 c milk (cow's or soy)	2 tsp coconut powder
2 tsp carob powder	2 tbsp soy milk powder
1 tbsp protein powder	2 tsp honey
1 banana, mashed	1 tsp pure vanilla

Put all ingredients in blender, add 2 ice cubes if you desire it chilled more. Blend well and serve in freezer chilled glasses. You can vary this with using fresh fruit available in season, peaches, etc., or adding other health ingredients — raw wheat germ, brewer's yeast, sesame seeds, etc. Serves 2.

SESAME PINEAPPLE PROTEIN MILK SMOOTHIE

2 c unsweetened pineapple juice	2 tbsp soy powder (milk subs.)
½ c sesame seeds	honey to taste
yolk of 1 egg (optional)	

Place in a blender: ¼ cup sesame seeds and 1 c. pineapple juice.

Now blend the other ¼ cup of sesame seeds with the second cup of pineapple juice.

Add more pineapple juice to the mixture if needed. Add the soy powder for more creamy texture and extra nutrients, and add honey to taste. Serves 3-4.

ALMOND-PINEAPPLE PROTEIN MILK

1 c almonds	1 banana
2-4 c unsweetened pineapple juice	

Blend almonds with small amount of pineapple juice, then add pineapple juice to desired thickness.

Follow the same procedure for cashew milk or peanut milk.

"A strong body makes the mind strong."
—Writings of Thomas Jefferson

136

BREADS & GRAINS

HERBS TO SAVOR BREADS:

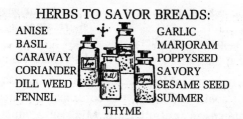

ANISE	GARLIC
BASIL	MARJORAM
CARAWAY	POPPYSEED
CORIANDER	SAVORY
DILL WEED	SESAME SEED
FENNEL	SUMMER
THYME	

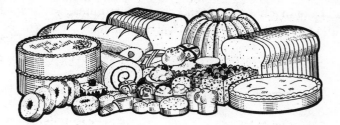

PUMPERNICKEL BREAD

Ingrid Klingler's

2½ c warm water	2 tbsp vegetable oil
2 squares fresh yeast	½ c blackstrap molasses
1 tbsp caraway seedts	1 tbsp honey
1 tbsp dill seeds	

Mix thoroughly, then add:

1 c branflakes	1-2 tbsp nutritional yeast
1 c wheat germ	2 c whole wheat flour
½ c soyflour	2½ c rye flour

Mix together, kneading about 5 minutes. Let rise two times then put into greased loaf pans.

Let rise again until almost double. Bake in 375° oven for 45 minutes.

BUTTERMILK CORNBREAD
Linda Barrett's

¾ c whole-wheat pastry flour
2 tsp cellu baking powder
1½ c yellow cornmeal

¼ c butter or vegetable shortening
2 eggs
1½ c buttermilk

Sift the whole-wheat flour and measure; mix with the baking powder. Sift again and stir in the cornmeal. Cut in shortening and add beaten eggs and buttermilk. Mix slightly just enough to moisten. Pour into a well-greased shallow pan, 8 inches square, and bake in a hot oven (425°) about 30 minutes. Cut in squares while hot and serve. Makes twelve to sixteen servings.

ALFALFA SPROUT BREAD

2 small potatoes with skins
1 quart water
½ c honey, plus 2 tbsp
1 tbsp Bragg Aminos
¼ c Soy Oil

1 tsp kelp seasoning
2 packages dry yeast
8-10 c whole wheat or Soy flour or combination of these
4 c 3-day Alfalfa Sprouts

It is important to use young sprouts; the older sprouts have a high water content and will make the bread soggy. Wash potatoes well, cut into small pieces and cook in 1 cup water until done. Liquefy in blender with 2 cups cold water. Put through strainer to remove skin particles. Measure and add enough warm water to make a total of 3½ cups liquid. Add ½ cup honey, aminos, kelp seasoning and oil. Dissolve yeast and 2 tablespoons honey in ½ cup warm water. Let stand 10 minutes and add to potato liquid. Stir in 5 cups of whole wheat or soy flour. Add sprouts, add additional flour to make a stiff dough. Knead well until smooth and elastic. Cover with hand towel. Let rise in warm place until double. Punch down and form into 2 loaves. Place in greased pans and bake in 350° oven for 1 to 1½ hours until well done.

BUCKWHEAT CORN MUFFINS
Bernardo's

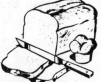

1 c buckwheat flour
½ c cornmeal
2½ tsp cellu baking powder
1 tsp Bragg Aminos

1 tbsp honey
4 eggs
1¼ c milk
¼ c unsalted butter, melted

Preheat oven to 400°. Mix together the buckwheat flour, cornmeal, baking powder, Bragg Aminos and honey.

Combine the eggs, milk and butter and stir into the dry ingredients until just moistened (batter will be thin).

Fill muffin tins ⅔ full and bake 15-20 minutes or until done.

HI-PROTEIN WHEAT GERM PANCAKES

6 eggs
5 tbsp cottage cheese
1 c raw wheat germ

½ tsp pure vanilla
1 tbsp unsalted butter

Put the eggs, cottage cheese, wheat germ and vanilla into an electric blender and blend 30 seconds.

Heat the butter in a 10-inch heavy skillet. Pour in the egg mixture and cook over medium heat until brown on the bottom; turn and brown the other side.

Serve with honey.

HONEY NUT BREAD
Doreen Fenwick's

2 tbsp butter or vegetable shortening
1 c honey
¾ c orange juice
2½ c whole-wheat pastry flour

3 tsp cellu baking powder (obtainable Health Store)
¾ c chopped walnuts
1 egg, well beaten
grated rind of 1 orange

Cream shortening; stir in honey and mix well. Add egg and orange rind; beat until creamy. Mix and sift whole-wheat flour, baking powder, and add walnuts. Add flour mixture and orange juice alternately to first mixture. Bake in a greased oven-proof glass loaf pan in moderate oven (350° F.) about 1 hour. This is better the second day. Makes 1 loaf.

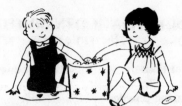

The recipe I am now going to give you is one enjoyed equally by both children and adults. I would serve this snack at times when my children, their friends and parents, were at our swimming pool for an afternoon of fun and it never failed to bring delight. I would make it up ahead of time by the gallon and towards mid-afternoon would set out a big party bowl of this delightful protein cereal mix. Along with it I would serve fresh fruit punch sweetened with honey and made with all natural fruits.

This recipe can be served at potluck dinners, birthday parties or taken on camping trips or long automobile trips. It is not only a delicious combination of foods but is a powerhouse of natural proteins. This recipe is delicious as a cold cereal served with sesame, soy or almond milk, and topped with fresh fruit.

HI-PROTEIN CEREAL MIX SNACK

Mix lightly in a bowl:

3 qts oatmeal	½ c soy flour
1 c natural cornmeal	½ c unsweetened coconut
½ c raw wheat germ	

¾ c sunflower meal or any nut meal such as almond, cashew or Brazil*

1 c chopped nuts such as peanuts, walnuts or pecans

¾ c chopped unsulphured dates

½ c sun-dried seedless unsulphured raisins

½ c seeds such as pumpkin, sesame or sunflower

Then mix:

½ c Bragg date sweetner	⅔ c raw honey
1½ c water	1⅓ c sesame seed oil

*First, make nut meal by blending whole nuts in blender.

Then combine all ingredients together. The mixture should be crumbly, moist and chunky. If too moist, add more oatmeal. Spread on cookie sheets. Bake one hour in 225° oven or until mixture is light golden brown. Yield: about one gallon.

SUNFLOWER AND SESAME MEAL
ADDS PROTEIN TO OTHER FOODS

Sunflower and sesame seed meal being a very rich protein source is an ideal way to fortify your meals with protein. Delicious when sprinkled over casseroles, salads, soups and vegetables. It is best when ground fresh in either a blender or a small electric mill. This way it retains the full goodness until you are ready to use it.

BAKED MILLET

2 tbsp Soy Oil	½ tsp rubbed sage
½ Onion, chopped	4 c vegetable broth
½ c fresh mushrooms, chopped	or water
1 c hulled millet	1 tbsp Bragg Aminos

Heat Soy Oil in a large skillet or saucepan. Add onion and mushrooms and cook until mushrooms are lightly browned. Add millet and cook and stir until well coated with oil. Add sage and broth. Bring to a boil. Turn into a greased 2-quart baking dish. Cover tightly and bake in 300° oven for 1½ hours. This makes a main dish when served with stewed dried beans or peas. May be served hot with poultry, fish or eggs if you desire.

CHEESE CRACKERS

2 c grated sharp Cheddar cheese	Dash of cayenne pepper
	Dash of Bragg Aminos
½ c unsalted butter	2 c whole wheat flour
1 medium onion (liquified in blender)	2 tbsp caraway seed

Cream butter and cheese together with electric hand mixer. Add onion, pepper, Bragg Aminos and caraway. Mix well. Work in flour until well blended. Knead the dough on board until smooth. Roll into long roll (or rolls) about one inch in diameter.

Chill about 1½ hours. Slice thin with sharp knife and place on baking sheet. Bake in moderate oven 350° for 10-12 minutes.

BUCKWHEAT OR KASHA CUTLETS

1 tbsp oil
½ onion, chopped
1 egg, lightly beaten
2 c cooked kasha (buckwheat groats)
1 tbsp chopped sunflower seeds or nuts

1 tbsp Bragg Aminos
1 tsp Bragg Instant
   Vegetable Broth Powder

Lightly saute the onion in the oil. Add the onion to the kasha, eggs, Bragg Aminos, Bragg Broth Powder, and the seeds or nuts.

Form into patties or drop by tbsp onto heated skillet. Saute over low heat until both sides are nicely browned.

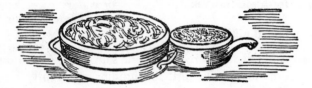

BUCKWHEAT GROATS (KASHA)
Chad's

1 c buckwheat groats
   (grains)
1 tbsp unsalted butter
¼ tsp Bragg Feast of the Sea (kelp)

½ tsp Bragg Aminos
2 medium eggs
2 c boiling water

Bring water to boil in separate pot. Heat up large frying pan with no shortening. Mix buckwheat groats and eggs thoroughly. Put into heated pan and stir until toasted. Grains will separate when ready.

Pour in 2 cups actively boiling water, add butter, Bragg Aminos and Bragg Feast of the Sea and stir thoroughly. Cover and simmer on low heat 12-15 minutes, until water is absorbed.

As a side dish will serve 4 to 6. For a complete meal, cut 1 medium tomato into small pieces and mix in groats after cooked. Top with 2 oz grated Natural Cheese and chopped parsley. Will serve 2.

SANDWICHES AND FILLINGS

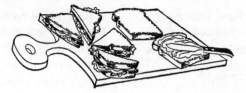

PEANUT BUTTER AND RAISIN SANDWICH

Wash and chop or grind ½ cup raisins. Combine with ½ cup peanut butter, adding enough orange-blossom honey to moisten. Makes 6 sandwiches.

CELERY AND PEANUT BUTTER SANDWICH

Combine ⅓ cup chopped celery, ½ cup peanut butter, 2 tablespoons health mayonnaise dressing. Makes 6 sandwiches.

COTTAGE CHEESE AND VEGETABLE SANDWICH

Combine ½ cup cottage cheese, 3 tablespoons radishes, chopped fine, 3 tablespoons celery, chopped fine, 3 tablespoons cucumber, chopped fine. Season with kelp, garlic powder, paprika, 1 tablespoon mayonnaise. Mix until well blended. Makes 4 sandwiches.

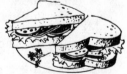

EGG AND OLIVE SANDWICH

Chop 3 hard-cooked eggs, and add kelp seasoning, ⅛ teaspoon paprika, and 12 sliced ripe olives. Mix 2 tablespoons of health mayonnaise and 1 tablespoon of lemon juice, and add to egg and olive mixture. Toss together lightly. Makes 4 sandwiches.

SLICED EGG AND CUCUMBER SANDWICH

Slice 3 hard-cooked eggs. Combine ¼ cup lemon juice, 1 tablespoon of cider vinegar, 1 tablespoon water, ⅓ teaspoon kelp seasoning and 16 to 20 thin slices of cucumber. Let cucumbers stand about 30 minutes. Spread whole-wheat or rye toast with health mayonnaise. Arrange cucumbers and eggs, season as desired. Top with lettuce leaves spread with mayonnaise. Makes 4 sandwiches.

CHEDDAR CHEESE AND GRATED CARROT SANDWICH

Crumble ¼ cup natural cheddar cheese with health mayonnaise and add ¼ cup grated carrots. Makes 3 sandwiches.

CHOPPED RAW CARROT AND RAISIN SANDWICH

Grate 2 raw carrots fine. Add 2 tablespoons chopped raisins, and add enough health mayonnaise to moisten. Makes 2 sandwiches.

CREAM CHEESE AND NUT SANDWICH

1 c cream cheese   ⅓ c minced nut meats
1 onion, sliced   1 tomatoe, sliced

Mix and spread on whole-wheat toast or crackers. Add tomatoes, onions and lettuce. Makes 6 sandwiches.

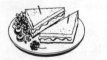

BANANA SANDWICH

Spread 2 thin slices of toast with butter, and lay on strips of well-ripened bananas. Add a bit of honey and a little lemon juice if desired.

PEANUT BUTTER AND BANANA SANDWICH

½ c peanut butter   1 banana
4 lettuce leaves

Mash banana and work into peanut butter. Honey or mayonnaise may be added. Top with lettuce leaves. Makes 4 sandwiches.

DATE NUT SANDWICH

2 c pitted dates   1 c chopped nuts
¼ c pineapple juice   lettuce

Put dates and nuts through grinder. Mix well with pineapple juice. Makes 6 sandwiches.

FAMOUS ROQUEFORT CHEESE SANDWICH

Blend equal parts of Roquefort cheese and cream cheese, moistened with a little softened butter or health mayonnaise. Spread this on slices of whole-wheat toast and sprinkle with chopped watercress. Top with lettuce leaf.

SANDWICH LOAF

Cut loaf of bread lengthwise into slices ½ to ¾ inch thick. Butter each slice lightly with salt-free butter or health mayonnaise. Spread bottom slice with desired filling, cover with another slice and continue in the same fashion until loaf is complete. Fillings may be different if desired. Spread top and sides of loaf with cream cheese softened with cream or top milk. One loaf usually requires three 3-ounce packages of cream cheese and about ¼ cup cream. Chill loaf before serving. Garnish platter with lettuce, watercress, radish roses, tomato slices, etc. The top may be decorated with nuts, sliced olives, pimiento, strips of green and red pepper. Cut loaf in thick slices. One sandwich loaf will yield 8 to 12 servings.

SANDWICH SPREAD

⅓ c cooked soybeans,
  mashed
2 tsp lemon juice
  (more if desired)

1 c avocado, mashed
½ c cashews, finely ground
½ tsp Bragg Aminos
  sage and paprika to taste

Mix thoroughly and place in container and use as sandwich spread or appetizer dip.

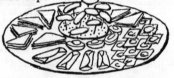

SPREADS AND FILLINGS

Bean Spreads: Combine cooked beans of your choice with chopped onion, minced parsley, health mayonnaise and make into a spread for dips, sandwiches or stuffings. When making sandwiches — substitute a lettuce leaf for topping instead of another piece of toast.

Egg filling: Combine 3 hard-cooked eggs, chopped fine parsley, a little grated onion, lemon mayonnaise dressing.

Date filling: Grind 1 cup dates and 4 tablespoons nuts using fine knife of food-chopper. Add enough orange juice to make the mixture of spreading consistency. A little lemon juice added will take away the too sweet taste.

Peanut butter and vegetables: Combine grated or ground raw carrots, celery, or onions with nut butter. Season to taste.

Tahini, soy or garbanzo spreads: Either alone or mixed are delicious and nutritious for sandwiches, spreads and appetizers.

Raw vegetables: Grind ¼ cup raisins and ½ cup each shredded cabbage, carrots, and apples. Add 1 tablespoon lemon juice and season to taste. Moisten with desired dressing.

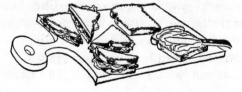

HEALTH DESSERTS
With Appeal for All Ages!

HERBS TO SAVOR DESSERTS:

ANISE	DILL WEED
BAY	FENNEL
CARAWAY	GINGER
CINNAMON	NUTMEG
CLOVES	POPPYSEED
CORIANDER	SESAME

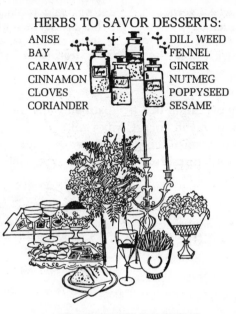

HI-PROTEIN GOODIES

Many people contemplating a meatless diet have a preconceived idea that this will deprive them of delicious foods. In this meatless cook book I am giving you recipes which I have tested in my own home and which have been tested by thousands of my health students. We find them to be delicious, nutritious and overwhelmingly tasty and healthful.

Since this book is concentrated upon obtaining generous amounts of protein, all recipes are slanted or originated to accomplish this purpose.

It was in Switzerland that Dr. M. Bircher-Benner gave me an outstanding protein recipe called "Apple Muesli". As you study the recipe you will see there is protein in the wheat germ, in the walnuts, and in the sunflower seeds—or you may use cashew nuts, Brazil nuts, pine nuts or almonds. To top off the protein, the recipe calls for ¾ c of yogurt.

APPLE MUESLI

2 tbsp old-fashioned
oatmeal
2½ tbsp raw wheat germ
juice of ½ lemon
¾ c yogurt
1 tbsp sun-dried unsulphured raisins (from your health store)

2 apples
2 tbsp raw honey
3 tbsp walnuts, chopped
(or any of the nuts or
seeds mentioned above

Soak oatmeal overnight in 4 tsp distilled water. In the morning add lemon juice and yogurt. Mix well.

Grate apples (unpeeled if organically grown and unsprayed) into mixture. Add remaining ingredients, mix well and eat immediately.

LINDA'S FAVORITE CUSTARD

2⅔ c milk
4 eggs
⅔ scant cup honey

⅔ tsp pure vanilla
nutmeg

Scald milk but do not boil. Beat eggs slightly; add honey and vanilla. Stir milk into eggs. Pour into custard cups and sprinkle with nutmeg. Place in shallow pan with hot water. When water comes to boil, place lid on top of pan for about 3 minutes. Bake to soft custard or until a silver knife comes out clean when inserted in center.

DATES AND NATURAL CHEESE

Dates are the oldest cultivated food in the world and are a storehouse of rich nutrition. Eaten with cottage cheese or any other natural cheese, dates make a quick and wholesome meal.

Be sure you buy only the natural dates. Your health food stores usually carry sun-dried fruits and natural dates. Commercial dates are mostly sugar dipped and added to this are preservatives.

ZESTY PROTEIN CONFECTION

½ c raw carob powder
⅔ c soy powder
2 tbsp safflower, corn oil or soy oil
¼ c unsalted peanut butter (from your health food store)

¼ c rice polishings
2 tbsp Brewer's yeast
2 tbsp raw wheat germ

Place all ingredients in bowl. Add enough raw honey to make consistency to knead. Spread in square pan. Press chopped nuts over the top. Chill and cut in pieces.

HI-PROTEIN FRUIT AND NUT BALLS

1 c seeded natural dates
1 c sun-dried natural raisins
¾ c natural unsweetened, unprocessed coconut

1 c raw wheat germ
1 c sunflower seeds, coarsely chopped
1 c sun-dried natural figs

(Note: All of the above ingredients may be purchased at your health food store.)

Put ingredients through meat grinder. Place in pan. Add enough honey to make consistency to knead. Spread in square dish. Sprinkle on natural unsweetened unprocessed coconut and roll into one-inch balls and refrigerate.

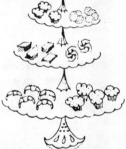

SESAME SEED PROTEIN DELIGHTS

½ c sunflower seed meal
¾ c Tahini (sesame seed butter)
½ c finely ground natural unsweetened unprocessed coconut

Mix all ingredients together. Separate into two portions. Place each on a piece of wax paper and form into a one-inch roll. Wrap in the paper and keep in the refrigerator. Cut into one and one-half inch pieces.

HI-PROTEIN CAROB BROWNIES

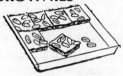

Have three sizes of mixing bowls.
Mix as follows. *In a large bowl:*

½ c honey	¼ c sunflower seed oil
2 tbsp blackstrap molasses	2 eggs separated. Beat yolks, add to mixture

In a small bowl. Beat the whites; set aside

In medium bowl:

½ c soybean powder	½ tsp. ginger (optional)
½ c sunflower seed meal	1 tsp cinnamon (optional)
½ c carob powder	1 tsp pure vanilla can be
½ tsp allspice (optional)	used in place of spices

Now add this mixture to large bowl, a little at a time. This will be very stiff.
Add:
½ c of chopped raisins or dates; mix well;
add the whites of eggs (beaten stiff but not dry).

Pour into oiled 9-inch square pan. Bake in oven heated to 350° for 25 minutes. Cool; cut into squares.

BAKED BANANAS

6 ripe bananas	3 tbsp honey
1 c pure freshly squeezed orange juice	1 tsp vanilla

½ c finely chopped walnuts or almonds
1 tbsp arrowroot powder (obtainable from health food store)

Mix well in baking pan the orange juice, honey, vanilla and 1 tbsp arrowroot which has been thoroughly dissolved in the orange juice first.

Place whole bananas in this mixture and bake in 300° oven for 15 or 20 minutes, or until bananas are medium soft. When serving spoon sauce over the bananas, adding chopped nuts.

FRESH BANANAS WITH HI-PROTEIN NUT BUTTERS

Cut bananas in half and spread on: cashew butter, almond butter, Tahini or peanut butter.

(Note: All these natural nut butters can be purchased at your health food store.)

PINEAPPLE SHERBET
Ingrid Klingler's

1 tbsp honey	½ c yogurt
1 sliced banana	2 tbsp fresh lemon juice
1 c fresh or canned pineapple, unsweetened	

Blend above ingredients and pour into ice tray. Place in freezer. When ready to serve, put through blender again until mixture is soft and creamy.

HONEYED APPLES AND RAW WHEAT GERM

2 pounds tart apples	1 c raw wheat germ
1 c honey	

Wash and core apples. Cut in quarters. In stewing pan allow honey to boil. Drop fruit 1 piece at a time. Continue cooking until fruit is clear. When serving sprinkle on generous amounts of raw wheat germ.

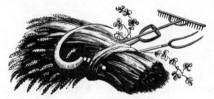

HI-PROTEIN YOGURT, NUT, WHEAT GERM MIX

Place 3 tbsp yogurt in deep dish. Sprinkle generously with raw wheat germ. Add chopped cashew nuts or cashew nut meal and honey to taste.

QUICK PICK-UP PROTEIN SWEETS

¾ lb natural sun-dried
    raisins
¾ lb natural sun-dried
    figs
½ lb walnut meats

1 tsp Brewer's yeast
¾ lb cashew nuts
¾ lb pitted dates
½ c sesame seeds
1 c raw wheat germ

Note: These ingredients can be purchased at health food stores.

Prepare the fruit by removing the seeds and stem ends. Put the fruit and nuts through a meat grinder with the coarsest cutter. Roll out the material on a board until it is about ¾ inch thickness. Roll it with sesame seeds and cut into squares.

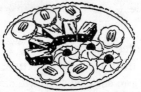

HI-PROTEIN BRAN WHEAT GERM FRUIT BAR

¼ lb pitted dried
    prunes
¼ lb natural dates
¼ lb natural figs
¼ lb unsulphured
    seedless raisins

¼ c honey
3 tbsp lemon juice
1 c bran
½ c raw wheat germ
1 tbsp grated orange rind

Note: These ingredients can be purchased at health food stores.

Grind fruit in food chopper, using the coarse grinder. Mix it with the other ingredients. Mold the mixture in a pan. Refrigerate 1 hour. Cut into small bars.

CUSTARD

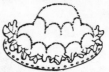

Custard is a splendid protein food and makes an ideal dessert. Here is the basic custard recipe:

1 c milk	1 egg or 5 eggs to 1 qt
2 tbsp raw honey	¾ tsp cinnamon
1 tsp pure vanilla	½ tsp nutmeg

Note: Eggs have a great deal to do with the consistency of custard. Use a smaller number of eggs when a thin delicate or soft custard is desired. For most custards, 1 egg to 1 c milk is about right.

When 2 egg yokes are substituted for 1 egg, it makes a smooth finer grained custard.

Scald milk. Beat eggs just enough to mix (too much beating makes a porous custard). Add vanilla and honey. Pour milk gradually over egg mixture, stirring constantly. Sprinkle spices on top.

Set baking dish in a pan of hot water and bake at low temperature (about 300°). Above all things, be sure water surrounding custard does not boil. Bake until firm or until inserted silver knife blade comes out clean. Remove immediately from oven. Watch carefully to avoid over-cooking.

DATE AND BROWN RICE PUDDING

¾ c chopped dates	4 eggs, well-beaten
3 c milk, warmed	3½ tbsp honey
1 c cooked brown rice	

Mix all ingredients well and pour into custard cups. Place cups in pan of hot water and bake in quick oven until set.

RAISIN AND BROWN RICE PUDDING

Follow recipe for DATE AND BROWN RICE PUDDING, substituting raisins for dates.

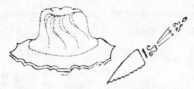

HI-PROTEIN CARROT PUDDING

1 c pitted dates
1 c raisins
3½ c grated, raw carrots

½ c honey
½ c cold-pressed oil
1 c walnuts

Put carrots, raisins, dates and nuts through food chopper. Add honey and oil, and pack in casserole. Bake ½ hr. in moderate oven.

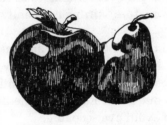

BAKED APPLES WITH WALNUTS AND HONEY

4 baking apples, cored
1 tsp cinnamon
4 tbsp honey

¾ c sweetened pineapple juice
⅓ c chopped walnuts

Pre-heat oven to 350°. Place apples in a covered dish. Stuff the apples with chopped walnut meats allowing a tbsp of honey for each apple to be poured over the walnuts. Pour pineapple juice over apples. Powder apples with cinnamon. Bake 40 minutes or until done. Cool and serve.

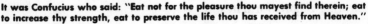

It was Confucius who said: "Eat not for the pleasure thou mayest find therein; eat to increase thy strength, eat to preserve the life thou has received from Heaven."

154

HI-PROTEIN RAW NUT ICE CREAM

½ c sunflower seed kernels	2 c milk
½ c sesame seeds	1 c almonds
½ c honey	1 c pecans
¼ c corn oil	

Mix all the ingredients together and blend in an electric blender in batches until it has a smooth consistency. Pour this mixture into ice cube trays and freeze until solid.

HI-PROTEIN NO-CHOCOLATE CONFECTION

2 tbsp carob powder	⅛ tsp cinnamon
1 envelope unflavored gelatin	½ tsp pure vanilla
	½ c chopped walnuts
¾ c water	

In a saucepan, mix together cinnamon and carob powder. Add the milk slowly to saucepan on top of stove. Stir constantly. Then add ½ c water.

In another cup, soften gelatin in ¼ c water; add to the hot candy mixture and stir until dissolved. Remove from stove top and add vanilla. Cool and as it hardens, stir in walnuts. Turn into buttered tin. Refrigerate.

HI-PROTEIN HONEY ICE CREAM

2 eggs, lightly beaten	¾ c honey
2 c milk	2 c heavy cream
1 tbsp unflavored gelatin	2 tbsp pure vanilla
2 tbsp arrowroot powder	½ c non-fat milk dry solids

In a saucepan, place the milk, eggs, gelatin, arrowroot and honey. Bring to a boil, stirring until mixture thickens.

Cool mixture. Stir in the cream, vanilla and milk solids. Mix well. Pour into two freezer trays and freeze about 1½ hours until mixture is frozen at least one-inch from the edges.

Transfer mixture to a mixing bowl and beat until smooth. (An electric blender can be used instead of an electric mixer.

Return the mixture to freezer trays and freeze again.

THE BRAGG TRAVEL DIET

In my lecture work, I travel all over the world in airplanes. Some trips are longer than others. When I make a long trip, I prepare a meatless meal of three or four different food items. On a short trip where I'll be eating only one meal on the plane, I carry a bag of sun-dried, unsulphured fruits such as raisins, figs, or dates, and with it I will have sunflower seeds, almonds, walnuts, Brazil nuts, cashew nuts or peanuts.

While the menus on the plane may satisfy the average eater, most of the meals are the standard restaurant variety using refined white bread, salted butter, frozen vegetables (I do not eat frozen vegetables), rich sugary desserts, coffee, tea and alcoholic beverages. This may be very nice food—but as a health minded person, it isn't my kind of food.

So on long or short plane trips or on busses or ships, I carry in my flight bag a variety of meatless foods which are very satisfying and nourishing to me. *I never compromise at any time as my goal in life is to attain perfection in health. If I cannot obtain my own meatless food, I'll fast until I can locate foods which agree with my philosophy of natural eating.*

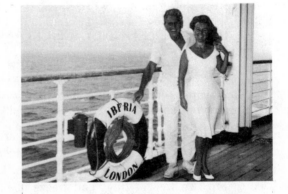

PAUL BRAGG and DAUGHTER PATRICIA
Travel the World Gathering Health Recipes

Many people who are interested in good nutrition will make compromises by eating food in airplanes, restaurants, and ships, thereby sacrificing their health principles simply to satisfy an appetite. This I do not do. I live the natural nutritional way no matter where I am traveling, and again I state, if I can't get what I want to eat I wait until food is available that is going to bring me health, vitality and long life.

SICKNESS IS EXPENSIVE

The biggest item in the average American's budget after food, shelter, clothing and transportation, is medical care. It is also the fastest-rising component. Between 1950 and 1973, while the four leading items were increasing 200%, the cost of medical care was increasing more than 400%.

In 1950 medical care absorbed only 4.6% of the average budget; 23 years later it accounted for 7.5%. The nation's total health bill in 1973 was $70 billion, or $350 per capita.

Sickness is big business. In the U.S. $11 billion was expended for drugs, medical supplies and equipment. To put the $11 billion in perspective, it is roughly one-third of what American's spent in 1973 on new automobiles.

To figure how much money is lost by man-hours on account of sickness would soar to astronomical amounts. In 1973, according to surveys conducted, $2.9 billion was spent at the drug store counter without a prescription. Of this total, cough and cold "remedies" accounted for $619 million, headache nostrums for $600 million, and mouthwashes and gargles for $240 million.

He who has health has hope, and he who has hope has everything.
—Mecca

Don't injure your system by over-feeding it. Over-eating will kill you long before your time.

VERY LITTLE MONEY SPENT ON PREVENTIVE MEDICINE

Most individuals have the attitude that they are indestructible and can drink alcohol, coffee, tea, cola drinks, soft drinks, sugary drinks, smoke cigarettes, eat refined white flour products and refined white sugar products, including products such as bread, buns, rolls, cookies, cakes, pies, and can eat bacon, ham, lunch meats, hot dogs and foods loaded with chemical additives and preservatives and still maintain health. *You are what you eat* and, in my opinion as a nutritionist and biochemist, sickness will increase to a point where within the next thirty years we'll have a plague of malnutrition equal to the plague of flu in 1918, and that millions will be destroyed by unhealthy eating habits.

This book is written not only to free you from paying exorbitant prices for meat, but also to impress upon you the importance of living on natural foods with a preponderance of fresh fruits and vegetables, properly cooked vegetables, and the natural proteins as given in this book. Living close to nature and a natural health diet is the only hope a human has to be free from the bondage of illness and the shortening of life.

"GETTING OLD"—TRUE OR FALSE?

In the vernacular of the average person, you will constantly hear expressions such as: "As you get older, your eyesight, hearing, strength and energy decline"—or "Your physical problems as you grow older are due to aging."

I don't believe these statements. We can degenerate physically but grow old—never! There's nothing to grow old. No part of the human body is over 7 years of age. Every 90 days we get a new bloodstream; every 11 months all the soft tissue is replaced with new tissue, and in the approximate cycle of 7 years, all the hard tissue of the body is replaced with new tissue.

So when one makes the statement "As you get older", this is completely false as the body is constantly renewing itself. When you look at your face in the mirror, you're not looking at the face of a few years ago. When you look at your hand or your fingernails, you're not seeing the same ones you had seven years ago—or even a year ago.

We are constantly changing in body tissue and structure, and time is not toxic. Time is purely a measure and not a force. It resolves into your biological years and your functional years. If you do not build a body tissue with 100% natural foods, then you're not going to have 100% natural, healthy tissue. Tissue made with dead, demineralized, devitaminized foods is inferior tissue, and inferior tissue brings toxic poisons into the vital organs of the body causing disfunction or what we term ill health. You cannot expect the body to look, feel and function perfectly with tissues made from poor nutritional material. There is not the elasticity and flexibility that is found in a body made with natural foods. I don't believe that we are punished because we live beyond 70 years of age.

We cannot break natural laws, they break us! So many humans attempt to do this and nature punishes them, not for their ignorance or indifference, but by their abuse and total disregard for the body. You cannot expect to build a strong heart, and strong arteries that do not harden, and to retain unlimited energy with poor nutrition.

Let me tell you the story of John L. who is around 70 years of age. John and I were tennis partners for a good many years. John was a robust, powerful man and he looked upon my eating of natural foods with humorous contempt. He boasted how he could drink alcohol and coffee, and boasted that he could eat anything that agreed with him.

Today where is John L.? He is in a nursing home. He has had two strokes—the first three years ago and the second a year ago. Since the last stroke he has been bedridden, incompetent and senile. He no longer recognizes members of his family or me. In other words, this powerful so-called healthy man is now dying of several degenerative diseases. He has hardening of the arteries, his heart is weak, and his liver is only working to about 60% of its capacity.

I asked his personal physician what was his prognosis, and the doctor answered, "He has reached the point of no return—his vital forces are no longer restoring his health and it's just a matter of time."

I personally do not believe that old age is an illness. I believe the symptoms of old age are produced by our habits of living.

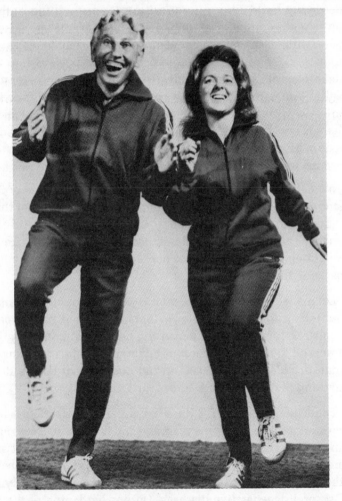

Paul Bragg and daughter Patricia carry out a vigorous morning exercise program faithfully every day, and keep in peak physical condition.

INDIVIDUALS CAN EXTEND THEIR LIVES
BY NATURAL LIVING

In various parts of the world there are individuals living 100 years or more, free from degenerative and debilitating illness. In a recent survey by the National Geographic Society, it was discovered that in the village of Vilcabamba in Ecuador, the small principality of Hunza in West Pakistan, and the highlands of Georgia in the Soviet Caucasus, there were people over 100 years of age living free of degenerative diseases. These people were physically active and healthy.

A census of the remote Andean village of Vilcabamba in 1971 recorded a total population of 819. Nine of the 819 were over 100 years old. The proportion of the population of Vilcabamba over 60 is 16.4%, as contrasted with a figure of 6.4% for Ecuador in general.

The valley that shelters Vilcabamba is at an altitude of 4,500 feet. Its vegetation appears quite lush. The people live by farming and their diet is practically a vegetarian one. Dr. Vela of the University of Quito, Ecuador, a nutritionist, found that the people of Vilcabamba consumed from 35 to 38 grams of vegetable protein daily.

In the surveys of the diet of the people of Hunza and Georgia, it was found that the people ate very little meat. Land is too precious to be used to support cattle; yet on this vegetarian diet, an unusual number of people far advanced in years appear youthful and have tremendous energy and agility to climb up and down the steep mountains of the valley. Tulah Beg, a 110 year old man in Hunza, is the champion mountain climber.

NATURAL DIET AND EXERCISE,
THE SECRET OF AGELESSNESS

The combination of a natural vegetarian diet and physical activity seems to be the miracle that keeps the people of these three nations in such fine physical condition at advanced calendar years. Natural diet builds strong body cells and prevents the accumulation of highly toxic material within the body.

161

Let's now consider physical activity. There is increasing awareness that in early heart disease we are paying for our largely sedentary existence. In the three areas I have been writing about, physical fitness was an inevitable consequence of the active life led by the inhabitants.

EXERCISE IMPROVES CIRCULATION TO ALL PARTS OF THE BODY

Through exercise, circulation is increased to the brain as well as to the heart and skeletal muscles. Recently it has been asserted that improvement in the oxygen supply to the brain will actually improve thinking.

Physical activity helps burn off excess calories and deposits of ingested fats and excess toxins.

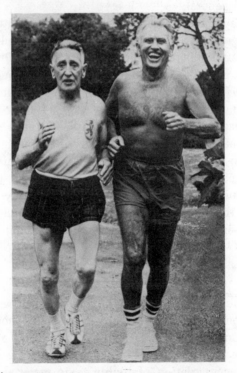

Paul C. Bragg (r.) and Duncan McLean, England's oldest Champion Sprinter (83 years young) on a training run in London's famous Regent's Park.

WHY SHOULD MAN DIE?

"Speak—write," saith the spirit. If one has anything to say for the betterment of his fellows, he should say it, and say it, too, in good, simple solid English. Here follows the warning—the ruin—and the remedy.

You are well today, reader, are you? "Yes."

Not an ache nor a pain in your entire body? "Not one."

Your health is perfect? "It certainly is."

Then were you to keep your health up to this present high standard, your body would not die, would it?

"I do not see why it should." Neither do I.

Think, consider again. Your body is now constituted of a number of atoms, a certain number of molecules and cells, and a certain number of bones, muscles, nerves, organs, functions; and many chemical elements.

Then you can positively state you are in perfect health? "I am."

Now, then, supposing that these organs, elements and constituents, were to remain in the same ratio of quality and quantity in your organism for years and ages, changing only for the better, if changing at all, you would not die, would you?

"I don't see why I should." Neither do I.

But, now, do I hear some critic say that these atoms, molecules, and cells necessarily wear out by use, or become impaired by friction? Yes, impaired or worn out to be replaced by others, and possibly by atoms and cells far more perfect and better adapted to such higher expressions of life as would greatly tend to the immortality of mortality on earth.

Seen in this light, there is no reason that man should die and should not enjoy eternal living.

Now I see the secret of the making of the best persons, it is to grow in the open air, and eat and sleep with the earth. —*Walt Whitman*

In health there is liberty. Health is the first of all liberties, happiness gives us the energy which is the basis of health. —*Miel*

"Everything in excess is opposed by Nature."

—*Hippocrates*

MAN NOT ORIGINALLY CARNIVOROUS

As discussed in some detail earlier in this book (See FRUITARIAN section), physiological evidence indicates that the human body was not originally designed for eating and digesting flesh. The formation of the teeth, the chemistry of the digestive juices, the length and structure of the stomach and alimentary canal follow a pattern similar to those of herbivorous (vegetarian) animals rather than the carnivorous (flesh-eating) species.

It would seem, then, that the eating of meat is an acquired characteristic of *homo sapiens*. It may have occurred during a long period of drought or extreme cold, when vegetation was unobtainable. Or early man may simply have experimented with flesh as food in imitation of predatory animals who sought him as a tasty meal. Who can say?

There are many theories of man as carnivore vs. man as vegetarian. From my own research and experience, I am of the opinion that the human being is naturally a lacto-vegetarian—and that meat, like salt (at a later date, to preserve the meat) is an acquired taste. *After all, more than 30% of the world's population never eat meat.*

Could it be that economics and environment—which probably influenced man to eat meat at sometime in ages past—are now influencing him to return to his original vegetarianism?

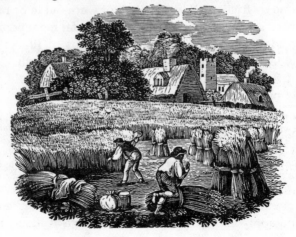

THE MEATLESS WAY OF EATING IS SIMPLE

Eating should be a simple procedure. You should never have to use a computer or to complicate yourselves with charts of vitamins, minerals, enzymes and nutrients to know what to eat, nor should you be concerned about the exact number of calories, grams of carbohydrates, and grams of protein in any particular serving of food. Then you make nutrition complicated and confusion takes the place of common sense.

Every human should eat freely and pleasurably to satisfy hunger—not to satisfy a numerical daily quota of nutrients. Most important, we should go to the dinner table relaxed and without fear of gaining weight. Eating should be a delightful experience, rewarding and guilt-free.

The meatless system of food selection is based to a large extent on the way people ate before food became one of the most lucrative and debased articles in the market-place. The meatless way of eating is sensible and simple.

People all over the world, for hundreds of thousands of years, have derived great pleasure from the simplest of meals long before nutrition was given the status of a science. Our ancestors of many generations ago ate when they were hungry without knowing a single thing about scientific nutrition. They selected and prepared foods the way their mothers and fathers did before them, and people enjoyed their simple food and were much healthier than we are today.

WHAT IS A BALANCED DIET?

Everybody is talking about diet and nutrition these days. The cry is, "balance your diet"—"eat right to keep fit"—"watch out for cholesterol"—"Beware of vitamin, mineral and enzyme deficiencies".

And the list of advice continues. From magazines, newspapers, television, radio, even from the cereal boxes, we are bombarded with nutritional information.

It is no wonder the confused housewife throws up her hands in helpless bewilderment. Who has the time to take care of a family and home, participate in community activities, and still read and apply all the nutritional knowledge available today?

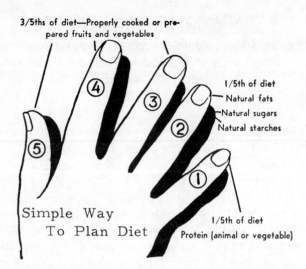

3/5ths of diet—Properly cooked or prepared fruits and vegetables

④ ③ ② ⑤ ①

1/5th of diet
Natural fats
Natural sugars
Natural starches

Simple Way
To Plan Diet

1/5th of diet
Protein (animal or vegetable)

EASY METHOD TO BALANCE YOUR NUTRITION

There is a simple way to bring order out of confusion. Let your nutrition be divided by five:

1. 3/5 of your diet should be raw fruits and raw vegetables, and properly cooked fruits and vegetables.

2. 1/5 of your diet should be meatless protein (50-75 grams daily). Sources include fertile eggs, milk and milk products, yoghurt, natural cheeses, soy beans and other dried beans and peas, lentils, whole grains, sprouts, eggplant, avocado, raw nuts and nut butters, raw seeds and seed butters, raw wheat germ, Brewer's yeast.

3. 1/5 of your diet should be divided into thirds as follows:
1/3 natural sugars such as honey, molasses, pure maple syrup, and dried fruit.
1/3 meatless starch such as whole grain flour, whole brown rice, dried beans and peas, potatoes.
1/3 natural fats such as unsaturated cold-pressed vegetable oils and unsalted butter.

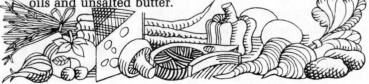

MODERN NUTRITION
CONFUSES EVEN SO-CALLED EXPERTS

Modern nutrition in the scientific sense has become extremely complicatd and confuses even professional people who should know everything about the right way to eat. Very few nurses, for example, know all they should about nutrition.

In my opinion, nutrition is simple. We should eat to satisfy the hunger within us, not the total of credits on some mental chart of vitamins, minerals, enzymes, protein, fats, carbohydrates, and calories. Personally, I believe computerized scientific nutrition is an almost complete failure, since hardly anyone has the desire or the patience to eat according to a table of numbers. Many people attempt to go on a good nutritional program but become so confused that they throw up their hands and return to their old habits of eating.

The result of our current food policy, based on supposedly scientific nutrition, has been best summed up by Ralph Nader.

"This country," he said, "is rapidly becoming one that has never produced so much food and so little nutrition."

The Bragg program works because I tell people to eat only food as close as possible to its original source, and to stay away from refined, processed, preserved and chemicalized food. In other words, make your diet simple, eat food that is natural, or close to its natural state.

By following this advice you can insulate yourself from many of the destructive changes that have taken place in our food over the past 75 years.

Much could be learned about simple eating by looking back at how people nourished themselves in earlier times. After all, the age of commercial food processing is comparatively recent—it has all happened in my lifetime.

"Tell me what you eat and I will tell you what you are."

To lengthen thy life, lessen thy meals.
Who is strong? He that can conquer his bad habits.
—Ben Franklin

I was born and reared on a large farm in Virginia. We grew practically all our own foods, had our own gristmill which ground natural grains; and people were not plagued with the mental and physical ailments of today. It wasn't until I entered a private school that I was introduced to institutionalized and refined, preserved, pickled, and other "junk" foods such as ice cream, cake and heavily sweetened desserts.

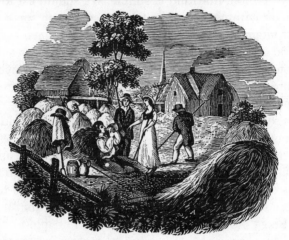

HEALTH WAY IS EASIEST AND SAFEST WAY

Eating the natural way is a simple and easy way to regain and maintain perfect health. For instance, let me tell you about how simple some of my meals can be.

I often make a lunch starting with a variety of raw vegetables, not even made into a salad. I slice some green cabbage, cucumbers, and half an avocado. Then I spread on cornbread either Tahini (sesame butter), peanut butter or almond butter, and finish the simple meal with a bunch of grapes, an apple, or a pear. Or instead of the cornbread and nut butter, I will have two hard-boiled eggs (mashed), with garlic and olive oil added. With this I will eat a piece of toasted cornbread. Of all the grains for making bread, I believe that natural whole grain cornmeal is nutritionally the finest grain one can eat.

Then again, I may finish my meal with a dozen almonds, some sun-dried dates, raisins or figs.

Another simple meal will consist of a prepared chopped salad with such vegetables as cabbage, carrots, celery and tomatoes, with a bowl of lentil soup on which I have sprinkled ground sesame and sunflower seeds. And I will finish the meal with applesauce.

Then again, I enjoy a sandwich meal. Between two slices of toasted whole grain bread, I will use mashed avocado, sunflower seeds, sliced raw mushrooms, lettuce and tomatoes, topped with a piece of natural cheese. I will finish this meal with stewed or fresh fruit.

When I have the time, I will prepare many of the recipes as given in this meatless cookbook, such as vegetarian patties, vegetarian loafs or cooked vegetables. In this meatless recipe book, I have endeavored to make the natural method of eating simple and delicious. None of the recipes are complicated.

Of course, you may not be able to adapt yourself to this system of eating at once, especially if you've just started studying natural nutrition. But read and learn, and gradually do the things your new health education tells you is right for you.

As you eat natural foods, you will develop an extrasensory perception for selecting what your body needs in the way of nourishment. I am in close communication with my body chemistry; call it instinct, call it anything you want, but my body tells me every day and every meal exactly what I should eat. Sometimes my body tells me to bake a potato, steam some carrots, eat some beans, cheese, or nuts. This didn't come all in a day—or a year. But now I can relate to my body's need for food.

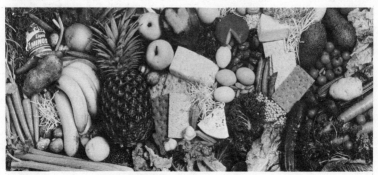

YOUR BODY IS YOUR CLOSEST COMPANION

"Know Thyself!" Be aware of your body's needs nutritionally. There is a still small voice within, with which you can communicate, and when this communication between you and your nutritional needs becomes a reality, you will move into a higher plane of physical energy.

After all, the greatest thing in life is energy. When you eat whole, natural food which is highly charged with solar energy, you then supply this energy to the living cells of your body. This is what we refer to as living on super-nutrition—always eating natural foods, foods that have locked within their cells unlimited energy from the sun.

As soon as you eat food which has been refined and processed, you lose the vital energy which that food once had. Let's take wheat, for example.

When wheat goes into a mill in the raw form, it contains the natural germ (rich in Vitamin E), liberal amounts of plant protein, iron, B-vitamins, and minerals. When wheat comes out of the factory in the form of refined white flour, it has been completely robbed of its mineral composition, its germ, its iron and the B-vitamins. Therefore, when you eat bread or other bakery goods made from this refined white flour, 90% of the wheat's potential energy is lost. Is it any wonder so many people suffer from malnutrition today when the food interests operate only in terms of profit, and not in terms of health? In my opinion, the tragedy of nutrition is the curse of civilization.

So before you eat any food which comes in a package, can or bottle, read the label. If it has been refined, if it has been preserved, if it has been hydrogenated, don't eat it!

When you eat natural food, your stomach won't cry out in an hour for more. People who snack all day long are suffering from malnutrition because their meals are not satisfying them, and we surely are a nation of snackers—ice cream, cake, candy, fried chicken, hot dogs, pizza pie, and other degenerated and defiled foods.

Whatsoever was the father of a disease; an ill diet was the mother.

—Herbert, 1859

Again I say, be aware of what you're eating. Before you put that food in your mouth, ask yourself: "Does this food contain the highest potential of solar energy which my body needs to keep healthy?"

Nutrition is an inside job and constant vigilance must be maintained in selecting food in our corrupt world today. Sometimes I feel that humans have a self-destructive desire to eat "junk" foods, regardless of the consequences. And so they pay a dear price with lost youth, lost health and years taken off their lives.

When you eat natural food, you'll be amazed how energetic you will feel, and how happy and fit it will make you. You'll be able to live on a smaller amount of food because the natural foods have locked within them this powerful solar energy of which you can avail yourself.

WHEN YOU'RE HEALTHY YOU'RE HAPPY!

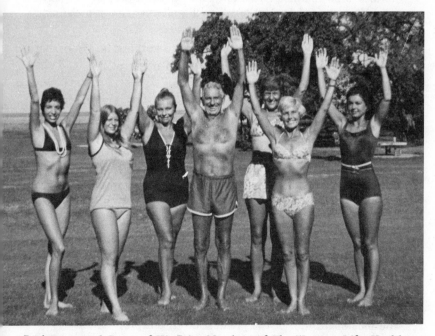

Paul Bragg and Some of His Prize Members of The "Longer Life, Health and Happiness Club" at Their Exercise Compound at Fort DeRussy, Waikiki Beach, Honolulu, Hawaii.

WHEN YOU ARE HEALTHY—YOU ARE HAPPY!
OUR PERSONAL MESSAGE TO YOU

When a person is motivated to change his life's pattern from the eating of "trash" foods to the eating of live foods, there comes to him an awareness of the great stride he has taken in joining hands with nature.

You have no security other than perfect health and that is the reason you must be constantly aware of what you eat and drink. You must be aware that you are protecting yourself against physical ailments of all kinds. You will control life and death in your body. You must be aware that you are now living in the highest rate of physical vibration—in a state of absolute "agelessness."

Every time you buy food, be aware that you are purchasing this food to increase your vitality, to immunize yourself by natural food against virus and infections. Be aware that each mouthful of natural food is going to make you a better person, physically, mentally and spiritually.

When you prepare food for yourself and others, be aware that you are doing it with loving hands; in other words, add the most precious of all ingredients—love.

You are what you eat. What you eat today is walking and talking tomorrow. If you keep this constantly in mind, you will not be tempted to eat "junk" foods. A mother with her two hands prepares for her family either Health or Sickness—make it All Health from today on!

In the spiritual ashrams of India, the most important monk is the cook. The cook must know what each monk requires to transcend into higher spiritual realms, that his body must be in the highest vibration. So in preparing meals, he must choose the ingredients that will revitalize the monks who have their feet on the pathway to transcendental living.

And so with you, be aware when you prepare meals that you are building health, strength, and agelessness, and that food is the master builder of the greatest of all temples—man.

From this moment on, be aware of the power of natural foods!

PROTEIN RESEARCH DATA

The meal planning pattern has long been built around a protein — rich food — the "entree."

The first recommended daily allowance for protein was high, approximately 130 grams per day.

1. Less Protein can Satisfy Body Requirements. Several food researchers "found that men could exist without apparent harm on intakes of protein from vegetable foods at a level of 30 to 40 grams per day; or 25 to 35 grams per day if one-third of the protein is supplied by animal foods." (L. Jean Bogert, Nutrition and Physical Fitness, 8th ed. [Philadelphia: Saunders].

2. Protein Excesses are Wasteful. A diet composed of too much protein leads to waste and possible injury to the liver because of the extra work required in the process of breaking protein down to a fuel food and excreting the waste.

"Each protein has an upper limit for utilization. Feeding more than that amount is inefficient and may put an excess burden on the organism to form and excrete organic compounds containing waste nitrogen." (M. L. Anson and John T. Edsall, "Advance in Protein Chemistry," *Biological Evaluation of Proteins*, ed. by J. B. Allison [New York Academic Press].

"What are we really doing to our bodies by giving them nutrients well beyond their needs as a result of our great fear of nutritional deficiencies? . . . To get rid of the additional protein means more work for the liver and the kidney, and these organs gradually hypertrophy to take care of the load." (L. E. Holts, "Nutrition in a Changing World," American Journal of Clinical Nutrition).

3. Vegetarian Diet Supplies Adequate Protein. The correct preparation of direct food crops (Non-animal, unrefined) will retain maximum nutrients and provide a vegetarian diet with an adequate amount of quality protein.

"African children suffering from protein deficiency disease responded as quickly when fed a combination of corn and beans (their native foods) as when given milk." (Albert S. Whiting, Report on treatment of Kwashiorkor victims, Muganeroe Hospital, Kibuye, Rwanda, Africa, 1973.)

173

PROTEIN and CALORIE COUNTER

This reference table is being included for those who want to use it. Almost every diet conscious person has become conditioned to checking calories and other contents of foods. However, I don't expect you to memorize these statistics, or carry around a mini-computer when planning your meals and marketing. If you follow the simple, basic rules which I have given you for a balanced diet, your own inner computer will program itself so that you will be able to respond to your body's nutritional needs without conscious calculation.

Foods are listed in average-serving amounts of 3½ ounces, unless otherwise specified. Listed for each food are: calories, amount of protein (in grams), and the amount of protein your body can actually use—U.P., or usable protein—if food is eaten alone, when these figures can be determined.

NUTS—SEEDS	Calories (grams)	Protein (grams)	U.P. (grams)
Almonds	598	18.6	
Brazil nuts	654	14.5	7.0
Cashew nuts	561	17.0	10.0
Chestnuts	194	3.0	
Coconut	346	3.5	2.0
Macadamia nuts	691	8.0	
Peanuts, roasted, with skin	582	26.0	11.5
Peanut butter, small amt. fat. salt	581	28.0	12.0
Peanut flour	371	48.0	
Pecans	687	9.0	
Pine nuts (pignolas)	552	31.0	15.5
Pistachio nuts	594	19.5	9.5
Pumpkin and squash seed	553	29.0	17.5
Sesame seed	582	18.0	10.0
Sunflower seed	560	24.0	14.0
Walnuts	628	20.5	10.5

MILK PRODUCTS—EGGS	Calories (grams)	Protein (grams)	U.P. (grams)
BUTTER			
1 pat	51	.0	
3½ ounces	716	.5	
CHEESE			
Blue (1 oz.)	103	6.0	4.0
Camembert, dom. (1 oz.)	84	5.0	3.5
Cheddar, dom. (1 oz.)	111	7.0	5.0
Cottage, uncreamed (1 oz.) ...	27	5.5	4.0
Cream (1 oz.)	97	2.5	1.5
Limburger (1 oz.)	97	6.0	4.0
Parmesan (1 oz.)	110	10.0	7.0
Roquefort (1 oz.)	111	6.0	4.5
Swiss (1 oz.)	104	7.5	5.5
CREAM			
Half & half (1 tbsp.)	20	.5	.4
Light (1 tbsp.)	32	.5	.4
Heavy (1 tbsp.)	53	.5	.4
EGGS			
1 egg (large)	80	7.0	6.5
MILK			
Whole (8 oz.)	161	9.0	7.5
Skim (8 oz.)	105	10.0	8.0
Dry nonfat milk solids (3½ oz.)	359	36.0	29.5
YOGURT			
Whole milk (1 cup)	124	6.0	5.0
Skim milk (1 cup)	100	7.0	6.0

BREADS—CAKES

Cracked whole wheat bread (1 slice)	60	2.0	1.0
Rye bread (1 slice)	57	2.0	1.0
Whole wheat bread (1 slice)	55	2.0	1.0
Cookies: Brownie (1 bar) (whole wheat)	55	1.0	1.0

175

LEGUMES—FLOURS—GRAINS	Calories (grams)	Protein (grams)	U.P. (grams)
Barley (natural)	348	9.5	6.0
Beans, white or red, cooked	118	8.0	3.0
Beans, lima, cooked	111	7.5	4.0
Blackeye peas (cowpeas), cooked	108	8.0	3.5
Buckwheat flour, dark	333	11.5	7.5
Buckwheat flour, light	347	6.5	4.0
Bulgur, dry (red winter wheat) ..	354	11.0	6.5
Chick peas (garbanzos)	360	20.5	11.5
Lentils, cooked	106	6.0	2.5
Macaroni, cooked (whole grain) .	148	5.0	2.5
Noodles, egg, cooked (whole grain)	125	4.0	2.5
Oatmeal, cooked	55	2.0	1.5
Peas, green, cooked	71	5.5	2.5
Peas, split, cooked	115	8.0	4.0
Rice, brown, cooked	119	2.5	2.0
Rye flour, light	357	9.5	5.5
Rye flour, medium	350	11.5	6.5
Rye flour, dark	327	16.5	9.5
Soybeans, cooked	130	11.0	6.5
Soybeans, tofu	72	8.0	5.0
Soybean flour, defatted	326	57.0	28.5
Spaghetti, cooked 8-10 min. (whole wheat)	148	5.0	2.5
Spaghetti, cooked 14-20 min. (whole wheat)	111	3.5	2.0
Wheat flour, whole	333	13.5	8.0
Wheat germ	363	26.5	18.0

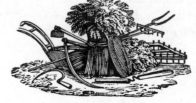

OTHER VEGETABLES	Calories (grams)	Protein (grams)	U.P. (grams)
Artichoke, cooked	30	3.0	1.5
Asparagus, cooked	20	2.0	1.5
Beans, snap, green, cooked	25	1.5	1.5
Beets, cooked	32	1.0	1.5
Broccoli, cooked	26	3.0	2.0
Brussels sprouts, cooked	36	4.0	1.5
Cabbage, cooked	20	1.0	.5
Carrots, raw	42	1.0	1.5
Cauliflower, cooked	22	2.5	1.5
Celery, raw	17	1.0	1.5
Collard leaves, cooked	33	3.5	1.5
Corn kernels, cooked on cob	91	3.5	2.5
Cucumber, raw	14	.5	1.5
Kale, cooked leaves	39	4.5	2.5
Lettuce	14	1.0	1.5
Mushrooms, raw	28	2.5	2.0
Onions, dry	38	1.5	1.5
Onions, green	36	1.5	1.5
Potato, baked in skin	93	2.5	1.5
Radishes, raw	17	1.0	1.5
Spinach, cooked	23	3.0	1.5
Squash, summer, cooked	14	1.0	1.0
Squash, winter, baked	63	2.0	1.0
Sweet potato	141	2.0	1.0
Tomatoes, raw	22	1.0	1.0
Watercress	19	2.0	1.0

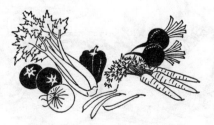

FRUITS	Calories (grams)	Protein (grams)	U.P. (grams)
Apples (1 small)	58	.5	
Apricots (2-3 medium)	51	1.0	
Avocado (half)	167	2.0	
Banana (1 small)	85	1.0	
Blueberries (½ cup)	47	.5	
Cherries, sweet (15 large)	70	1.5	
Grapefruit (half)	82	1.0	
Grapes (20)	69	1.5	
Lemon (1 medium)	27	1.0	
Melon (half)	66	2.0	
Nectarines (2 medium)	64	.5	
Orange (1 small)	49	1.0	
Peach (1 medium)	38	.5	
Pear (1 medium)	120	1.0	
Pineapple (1 slice)	52	.5	
Plums (2)	66	.5	
Prunes, uncooked (5 large)	172	2.0	
Raisins (½ cup)	200	2.0	
Raspberries, red (⅔ cup)	57	1.0	
Rhubarb, cooked with honey (½ cup)	190	1.0	
Strawberries (10 large)	37	.5	
Watermelon (1 slice) (medium)	156	3.0	

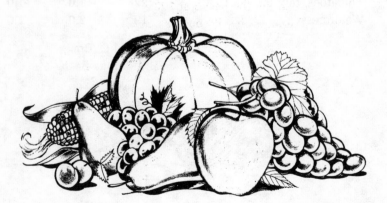

THE PEOPLE OF PLANET EARTH

When your knees begin to sag,
Straighten up and think of Bragg!

When your chin begins to fall,
Jut it out and think of Paul.

If you feel you're full of sores,
Crawl awhile on all your fours.

If you think you're courting death,
Give yourself the cleansing breath.

Stretch and bend, twist your aximus,
Do your homework, pinch your maximus!

Lungs and kidneys, heart and sternum,
Paul's got secrets, better learn 'em.

Belly in, head up, and SMILE!
Ragdoll, karate, dance awhile!

Exercise and fast and pray,
Come and live the "P.C.B." way.

Then, on the beach at 102,
Trim and fit—it could be YOU!

A Tribute to Paul C. Bragg
by Dr. Marcus Bach

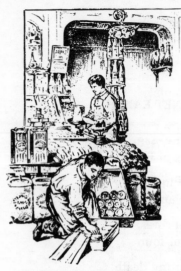

YOUR HEALTH FOOD STORE
The Specialist That Is Different

Unlike any other store, the Health Food Store is a specialist in Natural Nutrition. The people operating these stores are trained in the values of foods and can give you information in their factors and uses! Many people who have become acquainted with their Health Food Stores have gained knowledge that has given them a new lease on life . . . new interest that brings a great deal of pleasure and benefit.

The Health Store personnel are anxious to work with your nutritionist in offering you the foods he recommends and in helping you select foods that will stay within the limitations of the diet he has recommended for you. So be up to date in the field of nutritional science . . . read some of the books the Health Food Store has to offer you. The whole field of Health Food distribution was founded on idealism. It has maintained that attitude. You'll find pervading every store you enter, a sincere desire to help you get the most in the way of excellent nutrition.

Here are just a few of the featured nutritional health items:
- Bragg Aminos . . .
- Bragg Instant Vegetable Seasoning . . .
- Bragg Feast of the Sea (no salt) Kelp Seasoning . . .
- Bragg Date Sweetener . . .

- Bragg Mint Tea and Bragg Alfalfa Mint Tea . . .
- Bragg Natural Food Supplements for boosting your nutritional power . . .
- Whole grain cereals and products of all kinds . . .
- Natural sweetners, honey of all kinds . . .
- Natural Hi-Protein Meatless Foods . . .
- Date sugar sweeteners . . . raw sugar . . .
- Maple sugar and sweeteners . . .
- Bottled natural juices of all kinds. Fruit and vegetable . . .
- Jellies and jams sweetened with natural sugars . . .
- Coffee Substitutes • Herb Teas • Salt free foods . . .
- Fat free foods • Sugar free foods . . .
- Nuts of all kinds, raw and natural . . . nut and seed butters
- Sunflower, sesame, pumpkin seeds and others . . .
- Whole grain bakery goodies . . .

LET YOUR HEALTH FOOD STORE BE YOUR
MEATLESS BUTCHER SHOP

The Health Food Stores are stocked with hundreds of Natural Nutritional Foods for helping you feel stronger—look younger—and get more joy out of life!

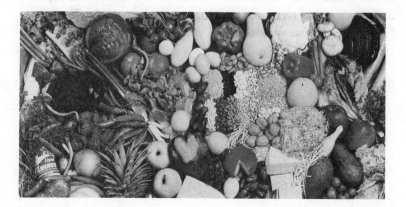

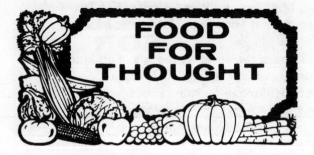

FOOD FOR THOUGHT

They who provide the food for the world, decide the health of the world. You have only to go on some errand amid the taverns and the hotels of the United States and Great Britain, to appreciate the fact that a vast multitude of the human race are slaughtered by incompetent cookery. Though a young woman may have taken lessons in music, and may have taken lessons in painting, and lessons in astronomy, she is not well educated unless she has taken lessons in preparing healthy meals. For women can either prepare health or sickness with their two hands. Proper nutritional planning is a must for the family. The right fuel [food] produces good performance.

The first wealth is health. — Emerson

Sir Isaac Newton, when writing his great work, "Principia," lived wholly upon a vegetable diet.

Hot-weather diet. — *The sultry period of our summer, although comparatively slight and of short duration, is nevertheless felt by some persons to be extremely oppressive, but this is mainly due to the practice of eating much animal food or fatty matters, conjoined as it often is with the habit of drinking freely of fluids containing more or less alcoholics. Living on cereals, vegetables, and fruit, and abstaining from alcoholic drinks, the same persons would probably enjoy the temperature, and be free from the thirst which is the natural result of consuming needlessly heating food.*

— Sir Henry Thompson

Behind the nutty loaf is the mill wheel; behind the mill is the wheat field; on the wheat field rests the sunlight; above the sun is God.

— James Russell Lowell

The wandering Arab lives almost entirely upon bread, with a few dates as a relish.

The world is moving so fast now-a-days that the man who says it can't be done is generally interrupted by someone doing it. — Elbert Hubbard

Get your happiness out of your work or you will never know what happiness is. — Elbert Hubbard

182

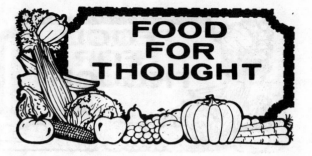

FOOD FOR THOUGHT

Soup rejoices the stomach, and disposes it to receive and digest other food.
— Brillat Savarin

To work the head, temperance must be carried into the diet. — Beecher

To fare well implies the partaking of such food as does not disagree with body or mind. Hence only those fare well who live temperately. — Socrates

The eating of much flesh fills us with a multitude of evil diseases and multitudes of evil desires. — Porphyrises, 233 A.D.

Health is not quoted in the markets because it is without price.

It is a mistake to think that the more a man eats, the fatter and stronger he will become.

The health journals and the doctors all agree that the best and most wholesome part of the New England country doughnut is the hole. The larger the hole, they say, the better the doughnut.

According to the ancient Hindu Scriptures, the proper amount of food is half of what can be conveniently eaten.

The nervousness and peevishness of our times are chiefly attributable to tea and coffee. The digestive organs of confirmed coffee drinkers are in a state of chronic derangement which reacts on the brain, producing fretful and lachrymose moods. — Dr. Bock, 1910

A physician recommended a lady to abandon the use of tea and coffee. "O, but I shall miss it so," said she. "Very likely," replied her medical adviser, "but you are missing health now, and will lose it altogether if you do not."

WATER

*To the days of the aged it addeth length;
To the might of the strong it addeth strength;
It freshens the heart, it brightens the sight;
'Tis like quaffing a goblet of morning light.*

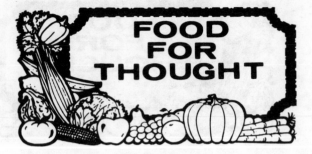

FOOD
FOR
THOUGHT

Fruit bears the closest relation to light. The sun pours a continuous flood of light into the fruits, and they furnish the best portion of food a human being requires for the sustenance of mind and body. — Alcott

The purest food is fruit, next the cereals, then the vegetables. All pure poets have abstained almost entirely from animal food. Especially should a minister take less meat when he has to write a sermon. The less meat the better sermon. — A. Bronson Alcott

There is much false economy: those who are too poor to have seasonable fruits and vegetables, will yet have pie and pickles all the year. They cannot afford oranges, yet can afford tea and coffee daily. — Health Calendar

The men who kept alive the flame of learning and piety in the Middle Ages were mainly vegetarians. — Sir William Axon

Hearty foods are those in which there is an abundance of potential energy.

If families could be induced to substitute the apple — sound, ripe, and luscious — for the white sugar, whiteflour pies, cakes, candies, and other sweets with which children are too often stuffed, there would be a diminution of doctors' bills, sufficient in a single year to lay up a stock of this delicious fruit for a season's use.

To maintain good health the body must be exercised properly [walking, jogging, deep breathing, good posture, etc.], and nourished wisely [natural foods], so as to provide and increase the good life of joy and happiness. — Paul C. Bragg

Statistics show degenerative ills increasing at alarming rates and attacking people at increasingly early ages. It is time the fact be recognized that diet is largely responsible for this increase, and that sugar, coffee, salt, refined and chemicalized foods, and the lack of exercise are the major culprits.

The lightest breakfast is the best. — Oswald

184

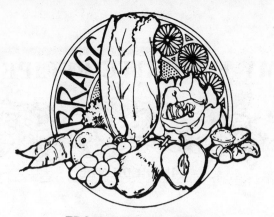

FROM THE AUTHORS

This book was written for YOU. It can be your passport to the Good Life. We Professional Nutritionists join hands in one common objective — a high standard of health for all and many added years to your life. Scientific Nutrition points the way — Nature's Way — the only lasting way to build a body free of degenerative diseases and premature aging. This book teaches you how to work with Nature and not against her. Doctors, dentists, and others who care for the sick, try to repair depleted tissues which too often mend poorly if at all. Many of them praise the spreading of this new scientific message of natural foods and methods for long-lasting health and youthfulness at any age. To speed the spreading of this tremendous message, this book was written.

Statements in this book are recitals of scientific findings, known facts of physiology, biological therapeutics, and reference to ancient writings as they are found. Paul C. Bragg has been practicing the natural methods of living for over 70 years, with highly beneficial results, knowing they are safe and of great value to others, and his daughter Patricia Bragg works with him to carry on the Health Crusade. They make no claims as to what the methods cited in this book will do for one in any given situation, and assume no obligation because of opinions expressed.

No cure for disease is offered in this book. No foods or diets are offered for the treatment or cure of any specific ailment. Nor is it intended as, or to be used as, literature for any food product. Paul C. Bragg and Patricia Bragg express their opinions solely as Public Health Educators, Professional Nutritionists and Teachers.

Certain persons considered experts may disagree with one or more statements in this book, as the same relate to various nutritional recommendations. However, any such statements are considered, nevertheless, to be factual, as based upon long-time experience of Paul C. Bragg and Patricia Bragg in the field of human health.

MY FAVORITE RECIPES

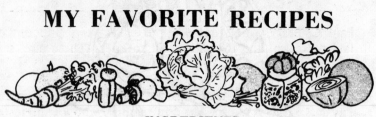

INGREDIENTS

SEND FOR IMPORTANT
FREE HEALTH BULLETINS

Paul C. Bragg, from time to time sends News Bulletins on latest Health and Nutrition Discoveries. These are sent *free of charge!*

The Health Builder, the magazine devoted to Nutrition and Physical Fitness, is also sent *free* to those who are interested in gaining and maintaining superb health!

If you wish to receive these *free bulletins* and The Health Builder — please send your name and also names of any friends and relatives you wish, using reverse side.

PLEASE SEND NAMES TO:

HEALTH SCIENCE - Box 477, Desert Hot Springs, California 92240 U.S.A.

name   (please print)

address

city   state   zip code

name   (please print)

address

city   state   zip code

name   (please print)

address

city   state   zip code

PLEASE CUT ALONG DOTTED LINE

Please send Free Health Bulletins to these friends and relatives:

Name

Address

City · · · · · · · · · · · · State · · · · · · · · · · Zip Code

Name

Address

City · · · · · · · · · · · · State · · · · · · · · · · Zip Code

Name

Address

City · · · · · · · · · · · · State · · · · · · · · · · Zip Code

Name

Address

City · · · · · · · · · · · · State · · · · · · · · · · Zip Code

Name

Address

City · · · · · · · · · · · · State · · · · · · · · · · Zip Code

PLEASE SEND NAMES TO:

HEALTH SCIENCE - Box 477, Desert Hot Springs, California 92240 U.S.A.

PLEASE CUT ALONG DOTTED LINE

BRAGG
Live Longer, Live Stronger
Self-Improvement
LIBRARY

*LET THESE AMAZING HEALTH BOOKS SHOW YOU
THE WAY TO A BETTER LIFE*

Each of these books is a priceless and valuable treasure
to help safeguard the Health of Yourself and Your Family.

__Hi-Protein, Meat-less Health Cook Book with History & Reasons $3.00
__Bragg's New Generation Health Food Cook Book 3.95
__The Miracle of Fasting... 3.00
__Building Powerful Nerve Force 2.25
__How to Keep the Heart Healthy and Fit 2.25
__Preparing for Motherhood Nature's Way 2.25
__The Golden Keys to Internal Physical Fitness 2.25
__The Natural Way to Reduce....................................... 2.25
__The Science and Art of Married Love 2.25
__The Shocking Truth about Water!................................. 2.25
__Your Health and Your Hair...................................... 2.25
__Healthful Eating Without Confusion 2.25
__Salt-Free Sauerkraut Cook Book................................. 2.25
__Beauty Book—The Hollywood Plan 2.25
__Nature's Healing System for Better Eyesight 2.25
__Building Strong Feet 1.25
__Super Brain Breathing.. 1.25
__Toxicless Diet & Body Purification 1.25
__Bragg Uses of Natural Cider Vinegar 1.25
__Building Health & Youthfulness 1.25
__Natural Method of Physical Culture 1.25
__Nature's Way to Health 1.25
__The Fitness Program With Spine Motion 1.25
__The New Science of Health 1.25
__The Philosophy of Super Health 1.25
__The South Sea Culture of the Abdomen 1.25

Remember, the gift of a Bragg book is a gift for life;

The books listed above can be obtained from your book or health store or directly
from Health Science. When ordering please add for postage and handling - 25¢ for
first book, 10¢ for each additional book. Remittance in U.S. funds only. California
residents add sales tax.

**HEALTH SCIENCE
Box 477, Desert Hot Springs, California 92240 U.S.A.**

Please send Free Health Bulletins to these friends and relatives:

PLEASE CUT ALONG DOTTED LINE

Name

Address

City   State   Zip Code

Name

Address

City   State   Zip Code

Name

Address

City   State   Zip Code

Name

Address

City   State   Zip Code

Name

Address

City   State   Zip Code

Name

Address

City   State   Zip Code

SEND FOR IMPORTANT
FREE HEALTH BULLETINS

Paul C. Bragg, from time to time sends News Bulletins on latest Health and Nutrition Discoveries. These are sent *free of charge!*

The Health Builder, the magazine devoted to Nutrition and Physical Fitness, is also sent *free* to those who are interested in gaining and maintaining superb health!

If you wish to receive these *free bulletins* and The Health Builder – please send your name and also names of any friends and relatives you wish, using reverse side.

PLEASE SEND NAMES TO:

HEALTH SCIENCE - Box 477, Desert Hot Springs, California 92240 U.S.A.

name   (please print)

address

city   state   zip code

name   (please print)

address

city   state   zip code

name   (please print)

address

city   state   zip code

PLEASE CUT ALONG DOTTED LINE

PATRICIA BRAGG, Ph.D.

Nutritionist, Beauty and Health Consultant

Advisor to World Leaders, Glamorous Hollywood Stars,
Singers, Dancers, Athletes

LECTURER and AUTHOR

Daughter of the world renowned health authority, Paul C. Bragg, Patricia Bragg has won international fame on her own in this field. She conducts Health and Fitness Seminars for women's, men's, youth and church groups throughout the United States . . . and is co-lecturer with Paul C. Bragg on tours throughout the English speaking world. Consultants to Presidents and Royalty, to Stars of Stage, Screen and TV, and to Champion Athletes, Patricia Bragg and her father are authors and co-authors of the Bragg Health Library of instructive, inspiring books.

Patricia Bragg herself is the symbol of perpetual youth, a living and sparkling example of hers and her father's precepts.

A fifth generation Californian on her mother's side, Patricia Bragg was reared by the Natural Health Method from infancy. In school, she not only excelled in athletics but also won high honors in her studies and her counseling. She is an accomplished musician and dancer . . . as well as tennis player, swimmer and mountain climber . . . and the youngest woman ever to be granted a U.S. Patent. An alumna of the University of California, and recently earning a Ph.D. in Health Sciences, Patricia Bragg is a popular and gifted Health Teacher.

She has been Health Consultant to that great walker, President Harry S. Truman, and to the British Royal Family.

Betty Cuthbert, Australia's "Golden Girl" who holds 16 world's records and 4 Olympic gold medals in women's track, follows Patricia Bragg's guidance. Among those who come to Patricia Bragg for advice are Clint and Maggie Eastwood, Connie Haines, Pamela Mason, Joe Feeney (singing star of Lawrence Welk's TV show) and his family of nine children, and Marilyn Van Derbur, the former Miss America who is now a famous TV personality, speaker and teacher. Patricia Bragg has helped many other official "Miss and Mr. Americas" . . . plus many thousands of unofficial Mr. and Ms. Americas and their families who read her books and attend her lectures.

From time to time, the Braggs send out startling New Discoveries in the field of Nutrition, Health, and Physical Fitness. Send your name, address and zip code for these Free announcements to:

HEALTH SCIENCE
Box 477, Desert Hot Springs, California 92240 U.S.A.